GOOD ENERGY COOKBOOK: UNLEASHING THE POWER OF ENERGETIC LIVING

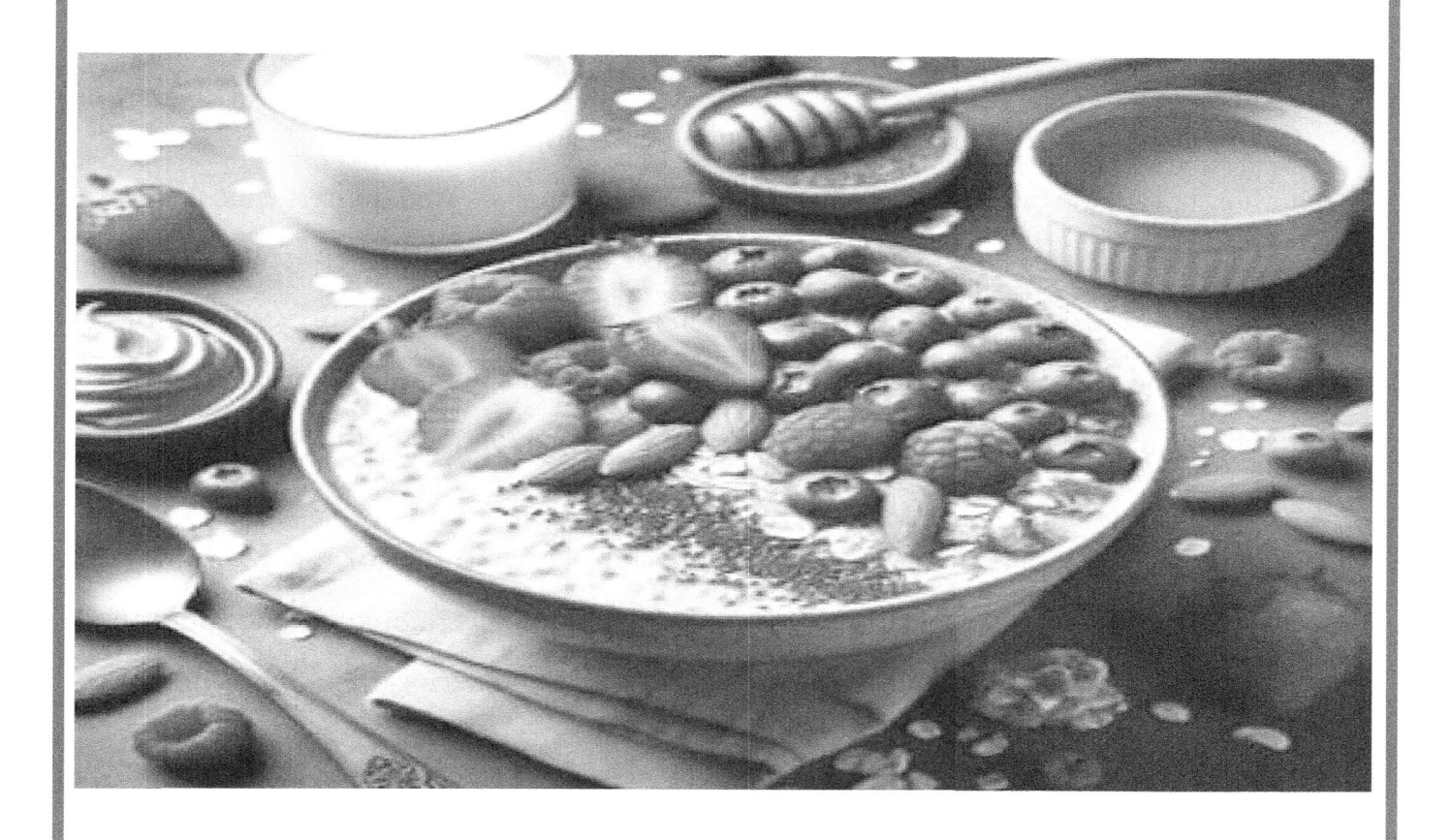

A Comprehensive Guide to Metabolic Health and Lifelong Well-Being Through Delicious Recipes and Practical Tips

Mary F. Thompson

COPYRIGHT

Copyright © 2024 by Mary F. Thompson

All rights reserved. No part of this book may be reproduced, stored in a retrieval system, or transmitted in any form or by any means, electronic, mechanical, photocopying, recording, or otherwise, without written permission from the author.

This book is a collection of recipes compiled by the author and is intended to be a source of inspiration, not a step-by-step guide.

All recipes and ingredients are provided as suggestions, and the author assumes no responsibility for any adverse reactions or outcomes resulting from their use.

The author has made every effort to ensure that all recipes and ingredients used are accurate and up-to-date. However, the author makes no representations or warranties of any kind, express or implied, about the completeness, accuracy, reliability, suitability, or availability respect to the book or the recipes and ingredients contained therein. Therefore, readers should always verify the accuracy of the recipes and ingredients before using them.

This book and its contents are protected by copyright law. No part of this book may be reproduced, stored, or transmitted in any form or by any means, including but not limited to electronic, mechanical, photocopying, recording, or otherwise, without the prior written permission of the author.

Dedication

To those seeking the limitless potential of health,

This book is devoted to those who begin on the incredible adventure of knowing and caring for their bodies. To those seeking vigor, high energy, and a life of infinite well-being.

In pursuit of health, each reader becomes a pioneer, traversing the complexities of metabolism and discovering the fundamental link between lifestyle and vitality. This devotion extends to individuals who aim for progress rather than perfection, believing in the transformational potential of educated decision-making and mindfulness.

This book is an homage to the tenacious spirits who confront problems with grit, the inquiring minds hungry for information, and the individuals determined to alter their lives using the concepts contained in these pages.

May the wisdom in these chapters inspire and lead you to a life full of positive energy, resilience, and the joy of living well.

With thanks for your dedication to health and our shared path toward boundless possibilities,

Mary F. Thompson

TABLE OF CONTENTS

COPYRIGHT 2

Dedication 3

INTRODUCTION 12

    The Relationship Between Nutrition and Metabolic Health: Unlocking the Body's Energy Factory 12

    Unlocking the Power of Food for Optimal Energy: The Blueprint for Well-Being 13

        1. Understanding Metabolism Basics: Breaking Down the Energy Factory. 13

        2. Balanced Meals for Sustainable Vitality: Nutrients to Fuel Good Energy Production 13

        3. Recognizing "Bad Energy" Foods: Identifying Causes of Metabolic Disruption 14

        Conclusion: A Blueprint for a Healthier, More Energetic You. 16

Chapter 1: 18

Understanding Metabolism—Navigating the Body's Energy Highway 18

    An Overview of Metabolic Function: The Energy Factory Within 18

    How Metabolism Impacts Health and Wellbeing: A Symphony of Cellular Harmony 19

        1. Weight Management: Balancing the Energy Equation 19

        2. Prevention of Chronic Diseases: The Metabolic Guardian 19

3. Mental Wellness: The Mind-Body Connection 20

4. Energy Levels: Unlocking the Power Within 20

Conclusion: Metabolism as the Conductor of the Orchestra of Life. 21

Chapter 2: 22

The Impact of Nutrition on Cellular Energy--Nourishing the Body's Power Plant 22

Building Blocks of Vitality: Nutrients that Fuel Good Energy Production 22

1. Carbohydrates: A Quick Energy Igniter 22

2. Proteins: The Cellular Architects and Repair Team 23

3. Fats: Sustained Energy Reservoirs 23

4. Vitamins and Minerals: Micronutrient Support Team 23

5. Hydration is the essential lubricant 24

Creating Balanced Meals for Long-Term Vitality: The Art of Culinary Harmony 24

1. The Plate Method: A Visual Guide to Balance 25

2. Snacking with Purpose: Micro-Meals for Sustainable Energy 25

3. Hydration Habits: Quenching Cellular Thirsts 26

4. Mindful Eating Enhances Nutrient Absorption 26

Conclusion: Fueling the Cellular Power Plant for Optimal Performance 26

Chapter 3: 28

Recognizing the Signs of "Bad Energy" Foods and Navigating the Dietary Minefield 28

GOOD ENERGY COOKBOOK: UNLEASHING THE POWER OF ENERGETIC LIVING

5

Identifying Foods That Disrupt Metabolic Health: Unmasking the Causes....28
    1. Refined Sugars and Processed Foods: Sweet Saboteurs 28
    2. Trans and saturated fats: The Fat Foes 29
    3. High Alcohol Consumption: A Metabolic Disruptor 29
    4. Highly and ultra-processed foods: the convenience trap 29

Strategies for Minimizing Harmful Dietary Choices: A Roadmap to Healthier Eating Habits 30

Conclusion: Navigating to Metabolic Resilience 32

Chapter 4: 35

Monitoring Metabolic Health Through Diet—The Power of Biomarkers 35

Use Biomarkers to Assess Nutritional Status: Decoding the Body's Messages 35
    1. Blood Glucose Levels: The Sugar Balance Indicator 35
    2. Cholesterol Levels: The Lipid Profile for Cardiovascular Health .36
    3. Inflammation Markers: Determining Internal Stress Levels 36
    4. Nutrient Levels: Assessing Micronutrient Status 36
    5. Hemoglobin A1c, the Long-Term Blood Sugar Gauge 37

Tracking Progress and Making Informed Dietary Changes: A Personalized Approach 37

Conclusion: Empowering with Knowledge and Action 39

Chapter 5: 41

Creating a Good Energy Meal Plan--A Four-Week Blueprint for Optimal Health 41

Developing a Four-Week Meal Plan for Optimal Health: The Architecture of Well-Being 41
    1. Assessing Nutritional Needs: A Personal Approach 41
    2. Understanding Macronutrient Ratios: The Building Blocks of Energy. 42
    3. Incorporating Micronutrients: A Nutrient Symphony 42
    4. Meal Timing and Frequency: Providing Consistent Nutrition for the Body 42
    5. Hydration: the Overlooked Elixir 43
A Sample Four-Week Meal Plan that Balances Nutrition and Variety 43
    Week 1: Breakfast, Lunch, Dinner and Snacks 43
    1. Explore Culinary Diversity: A Feast for the Senses. 45
    2. Mindful Eating: Enjoying Every Bite 45
    3. Adaptability and Flexibility: A Dynamic Approach 45
    4. Portion Control: Quality vs Quantity 46
    5. Social and Cultural Influences: Nourish the Soul 46
Conclusion: A Culinary Symphony for Long-Term Health 46
Chapter 6: 49
Principles of Good Energy Eating—Unraveling Dietary Philosophies for Lifelong Health 49
Understanding Dietary Philosophies and Myths: Navigating the Food Maze 49
    1. Low-Fat vs. Low-Carb Dilemma: The Macronutrient Battle 49

2. Myth about "Magic" Foods: No Panacea Exists 50

3. Detox Diets: Identifying Facts from Fiction 50

4. The Gluten-Free Craze: Navigating Sensitivities 50

5. Superfood Hype: The Truth About Nutrient-Rich Foods 51

A Comprehensive Approach to Implementing Sustainable Food Principles for Long-Term Health 51

1. Whole Food Focus: Accepting Nutrient Density 51

2. Moderation and Balance: Avoiding Extremes 52

- Practical Tip: 52

3. Individualized Nutrition: Recognizing Bioindividuality 52

- Practical Tip: 52

4. Mindful Eating: Enhancing the Dining Experience 52

- Practical Tip: 53

5. Seasonal and Local Choices: Supporting Sustainability 53

- Practical Tip: 53

Conclusion: Nourishing a Lifetime of Good Energy 53

Chapter 7 55

Improving Sleep and Circadian Rhythm for Better Metabolism: Unlocking the Power of Rest 55

Understanding the Relationship between Sleep and Energy Balance: The Sleep-Metabolism Nexus 55

Practical Strategies for Improving Sleep Quality and Rhythm: The Road to Relaxing Nights 56

Conclusion: A Symphony of Sleep and Metabolism 59

Chapter 8 61

Integrating Movement and Exercise for Metabolic Health 61

The Dance of Daily Activity and Purposeful Exercise 61

Embracing Everyday Activities to Increase Physical Activity: The Power of Movement 61

Creating a Balanced Exercise Routine for Overall Health: Purposeful Movement 63

Creating Your Personal Movement Symphony: A Lifelong Journey. 66

Conclusion: A Symphony of Movement for Metabolic Harmony 68

Chapter 9 71

Exploring the Benefits of Temperature Exposure 71

Harnessing the Power of Cold and Heat for Metabolic Resilience 71

Using Cold to Improve Metabolic Resilience: The Icy Path to Health 71

Safe and Effective Practices for Cold Exposure: Navigating the Chill. ... 73

Using Heat for Metabolic Resilience: Embracing the Warmth Within 75

Safe and Effective Practices for Heat Exposure: Embrace the Warmth 77

Conclusion: Embracing Thermal Symphony for Metabolic Harmony 79

Chapter 10 81

Navigating the Grocery Store for Good Energy Foods 81

A Guide to Making Informed Decisions in the Aisles 81

Making Informed Choices in the Aisles: Understanding Food Labels and Marketing 81

Tips for Selecting Nutrient-Dense Ingredients: Creating a Foundation for Good Energy Meal 84

Conclusion: Making Grocery Shopping a Positive Energy Experience ... 87

Chapter 11 89

Cooking Techniques to Preserve Nutritional Value 89

A Culinary Guide to Maximizing Good Energy 89

Maximizing Nutrient Retention via Cooking Methods: Unraveling the Science of Cooking 89

Recipes and Tips for Cooking with Good Energy in Mind: Enhance Your Culinary Creations 92

Conclusion: Infusing Each Meal with Good Energy 96

Chapter 12: 97

Recipes for Good Energy 97

Crafting Culinary Delights for Every Meal 97

Breakfast: Fueling Your Day Right—A Wholesome Start for Good Energy 97

Conclusion: Creating a Culinary Symphony of Positive Energy 105

Conclusion: 107

Embracing the Good Energy Lifestyle 107

A Journey to Empowered Health 107

Conclusion: A Call to Action for Lifelong Well-being 111

Glossary of Key Terms: 113

A Layperson's Guide to Understanding Good Energy and Metabolic Health 113
Conclusion: Navigating the Path to Wellbeing with Confidence 119

INTRODUCTION

In the world of health and wellness, the subtle dance between what we eat and how our bodies operate is a fascinating and important part that is sometimes neglected. This cookbook takes readers on a journey to discover the profound link between nutrition and metabolic health, providing a guidance on how to harness the power of food for maximum energy. Let's look at the complexities of this link, bringing down complex topics into simple words for anybody looking to improve their well-being.

The Relationship Between Nutrition and Metabolic Health: Unlocking the Body's Energy Factory

Metabolism, which is frequently seen as a mysterious black box, is the collection of activities that turn the food we ingest into energy that our bodies can utilize. At its heart, metabolism governs how effectively our cells make and use energy, playing an important role in determining our general health. This involves everything from keeping a healthy weight to avoiding chronic illnesses and improving mental health.

To understand this connection, envision your body as a smart machine with a complex energy plant within. This factory, known as metabolism, accepts raw materials (food) and converts them into useable energy, which powers every cellular activity, from breathing to thinking. The quality and amount of the raw materials we offer determine the effectiveness of this energy generation process, emphasizing the importance of nutrition in this complex system.

Unlocking the Power of Food for Optimal Energy: The Blueprint for Well-Being

Now that we understand how diet affects metabolic health, let us look at how we may use food to improve our energy levels and general well-being. It's more than simply counting calories or following rigid diets; it's about knowing the nutrients our bodies require to flourish and developing a sustainable approach to nutrition.

1. Understanding Metabolism Basics: Breaking Down the Energy Factory.

Metabolism may be compared to a factory with many departments, each responsible for a certain duty. Enzymes function as workers, breaking down food into its constituents—carbohydrates into sugars, proteins into amino acids, and fats into fatty acids. These building components are subsequently converted into adenosine triphosphate (ATP), the cellular energy currency, via several processes.

In simplest terms, think of food as Lego bricks. The body disassembles these blocks and reassembles them into the exact structures it requires. The more effectively this process operates, the more energy is produced for our everyday activities.

2. Balanced Meals for Sustainable Vitality: Nutrients to Fuel Good Energy Production

To power our energy plant optimally, we must supply it with the proper raw materials. This entails introducing a range of nutrients into our diet:

- **carbohydrates:** These are the principal energy sources, providing rapid fuel for urgent energy requirements. Choose whole grains, fruits, and veggies for long-term energy release.

- **Protein:** Proteins are essential for tissue construction and repair, and they help to provide a consistent and long-lasting energy source. Include lean meats, beans, and dairy products in your meals.

- **Fats:** Despite their negative image, fats are necessary for energy storage and a variety of biological processes. Choose healthy fats from foods like avocados, almonds, and olive oil.

- **Vitamins and Minerals:** These micronutrients work as metabolic catalysts, ensuring that the energy factory runs smoothly. Include a diverse range of fruits and vegetables to gain a variety of vitamins and minerals.

- **Hydrature:** Water is essential in metabolic activities, serving as a mediator for chemical reactions. Maintain appropriate hydration to promote effective metabolism.

3. Recognizing "Bad Energy" Foods: Identifying Causes of Metabolic Disruption

Certain meals can interrupt the smooth operation of our metabolic systems in the same way that certain materials might clog industry machinery. These "bad energy" meals frequently promote inflammation, insulin resistance, and other metabolic abnormalities, laying the groundwork for health problems.

-Refined sugars and processed food: These frequently cause fast blood sugar rises, taxing the insulin response and contributing to metabolic imbalances.

- Trans and saturated fats: These fats, which are commonly found in processed and fried meals, can cause inflammation and interfere with cellular function.

- Excessive alcohol consumption: While moderate alcohol use may offer health advantages, excessive drinking can strain the liver and impair metabolic processes.

Understanding these disruptors enables individuals to make educated decisions, avoiding items that may jeopardize metabolic health.

4. Metabolic Health Monitoring with Diet: Using Biomarkers to Assess Nutritional Status

Just as a factory manager checks output metrics, we may track our metabolic health using biomarkers—indicators that represent the efficiency of our energy factory. These indicators give crucial information about how well our bodies digest and use nutrition.

- Blood glucose levels: Monitoring blood glucose levels, which reflect how rapidly our bodies metabolize carbs, can help uncover possible insulin resistance or diabetes risks.

- **Cholesterol Levels:** High levels of LDL ("bad") cholesterol and low levels of HDL ("good") cholesterol may suggest an imbalance in fat metabolism.

- **Inflammation Marker:** Elevated levels of inflammatory markers, such as C-reactive protein (CRP), may indicate continuous inflammation, which can affect metabolic processes.

- **Nutritional Levels:** Regular blood testing may determine levels of key nutrients such as vitamin D, B12, and iron, revealing probable shortages.

Individuals may address imbalances proactively by monitoring these indicators on a regular basis and making educated changes to their food and lifestyle for long-term metabolic health.

Conclusion: A Blueprint for a Healthier, More Energetic You.

To summarize, knowing the relationship between diet and metabolic health gives a roadmap for nurturing optimal energy and general well-being. By understanding our bodies as complicated energy factories powered by the foods we ingest, we obtain insights on how to promote effective energy production. Individuals may take control of their health journey by eating a well-balanced diet, making wise food choices, and regularly monitoring metabolic indicators.

This cookbook is intended to lead you through this journey, providing not just recipes but also a thorough grasp of the concepts underlying effective energy production. As we progress through the following chapters, we'll learn how to create meal plans, analyze nutritional theories, and incorporate practical tactics for improved sleep, movement, and temperature change. It's time to accept food's ability as a catalyst for positive energy and set off on a revolutionary journey to a healthier, more energetic self.

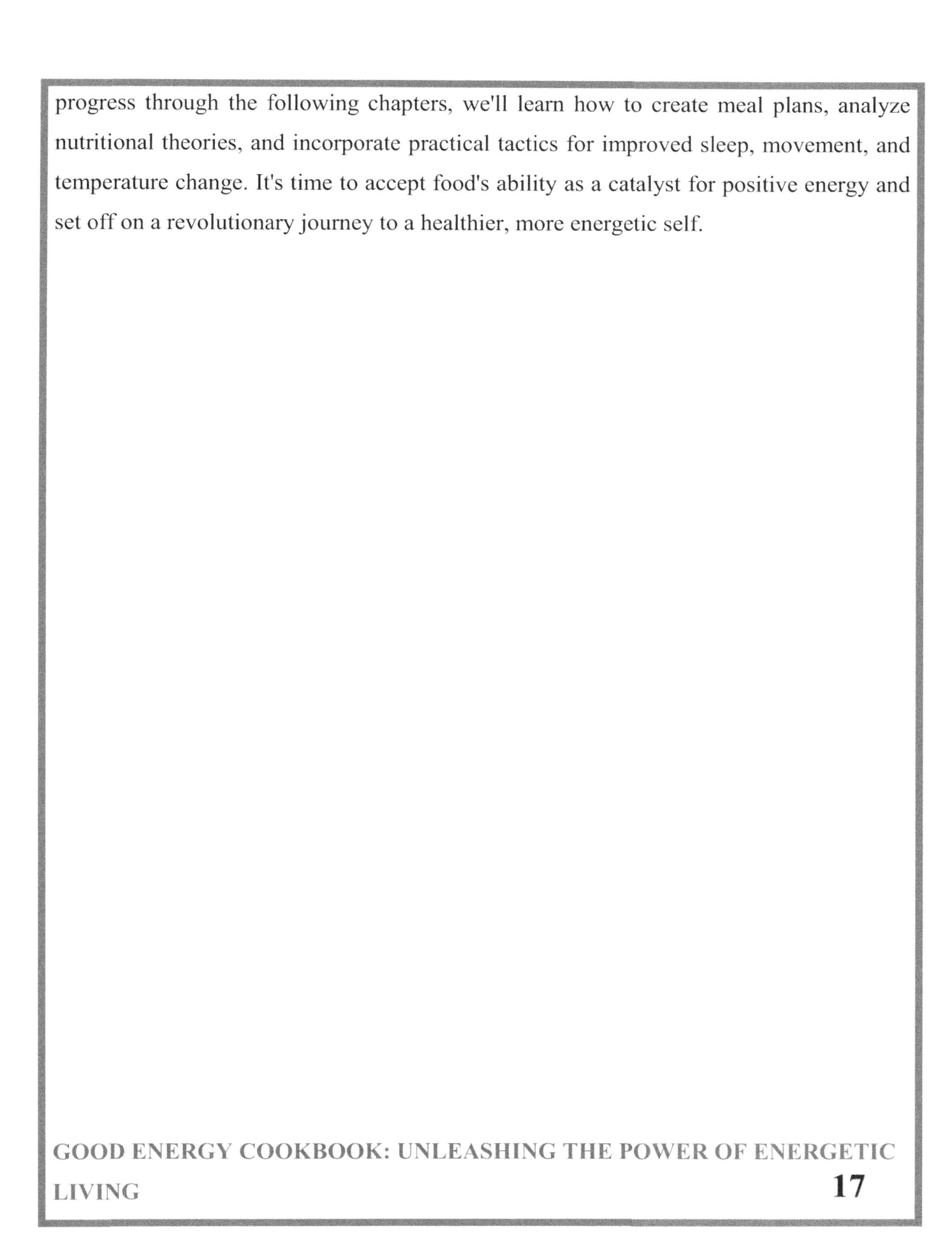

Chapter 1:
Understanding Metabolism—Navigating the Body's Energy Highway

In the complicated fabric of human health, the phrase "metabolism" frequently occurs as a mysterious power regulating our well-being. However, breaking down this complicated idea into manageable chunks reveals an intriguing mechanism that serves as the foundation of our vitality. This chapter acts as a compass, guiding us through the fundamentals of metabolic function and giving light on how metabolism affects our health and general well-being.

An Overview of Metabolic Function: The Energy Factory Within

Consider your body to be a busy factory that operates around the clock to satisfy the needs of daily living. At the core of this factory is metabolism, a sequence of complex chemical events that convert the food we ingest into the energy our cells require. Consider the food you eat as raw materials, similar to feeding a fire. As these raw materials move across the manufacturing floor, they are meticulously broken down, eventually creating energy in a form that our cells can easily consume.

To understand the fundamentals, imagine metabolism as a workforce constantly building and dismantling molecules. Enzymes work diligently, breaking down complex compounds such as carbohydrates, proteins, and lipids into simpler components. These smaller components then follow several routes, finally resulting in the production of adenosine triphosphate (ATP), the cellular energy currency.

How Metabolism Impacts Health and Wellbeing: A Symphony of Cellular Harmony

Now that we've uncovered the underlying workings of metabolism, let's look at how this complex symphony of cellular harmony affects our health and well-being. Metabolism is more than just creating energy; it's a dynamic process that is critical to preserving the body's delicate balance.

1. Weight Management: Balancing the Energy Equation

Metabolism determines whether we acquire, decrease, or retain weight. The energy we ingest from meals must be balanced with the energy our bodies spend via various activities and biological processes. If this equilibrium shifts in favor of excessive energy consumption, the excess is stored as fat. In contrast, when energy expenditure exceeds intake, weight loss happens. Understanding this delicate balance enables people to make educated diet and lifestyle decisions, promoting a healthy weight and avoiding obesity-related illnesses.

2. Prevention of Chronic Diseases: The Metabolic Guardian

Metabolism protects against chronic illnesses such as heart disease and diabetes. When metabolism is working properly, it regulates blood sugar, manages cholesterol, and keeps inflammation at bay. In contrast, changes in metabolic pathways can result in insulin resistance, elevated blood pressure, and a chain reaction of events that contribute to chronic diseases. Individuals might strengthen their defenses against these widespread health hazards by promoting metabolic health via prudent lifestyle choices.

3. Mental Wellness: The Mind-Body Connection

Metabolic health has an impact on mental health in addition to physical health. The energy created by metabolism powers the brain's processes, influencing cognitive functions, emotions, and even the ability to tolerate stress. When metabolism slows, it can lead to mental tiredness, mood fluctuations, and difficulties concentrating. Understanding the mind-body link emphasizes the need of sustaining both our bodies and our minds with a well-balanced, nutrient-dense diet.

4. Energy Levels: Unlocking the Power Within

One of the most tangible results of a healthy metabolism is consistent energy levels. Efficient energy generation ensures that cells have a steady supply of ATP, the essential energy currency necessary for all cellular processes. When metabolism is improved, people enjoy increased endurance, less weariness, and a general sense of vigor. On the other hand, a slow metabolism can cause chronic fatigue and a lack of energy, which can have a negative influence on everyday activities.

Understanding the enormous impact of metabolism on various areas of health provides individuals with the knowledge they need to make decisions that nourish this complex system, supporting overall well-being.

Conclusion: Metabolism as the Conductor of the Orchestra of Life.

To summarize, knowing metabolism is analogous to determining the conductor's job in an orchestra. Metabolism orchestrates the symphony of life within our bodies, ensuring that each instrument plays its role in perfect harmony. It is more than just a procedure; it is a dynamic force that determines the ebb and flow of our health.

As we've progressed through this chapter, we've looked at metabolism as a metaphorical factory, dissecting its basic activities and learning how it affects our health and overall well-being. Armed with this information, we are better prepared to navigate the twists and turns of our health journey, making educated decisions that enhance the harmonic symphony of our metabolic orchestra.

As we progress through this gastronomic journey, each recipe and nutritional choice becomes a note in the symphony, adding to the overall harmony of our metabolic orchestra. In the following chapters, we will dig deeper into the practical activities and lifestyle choices that may help us fine-tune our metabolic symphony and live a healthier, more vibrant life. So, let the orchestra play on, with metabolism as the conductor of our path to optimal health.

Chapter 2:

The Impact of Nutrition on Cellular Energy-- Nourishing the Body's Power Plant

Chapter 2 delves into the complex relationship between our food choices and the cellular processes that power our bodies, revealing the tremendous influence of nutrition on cellular energy. Consider our bodies to be complicated power plants, with food serving as the fuel that keeps them running smoothly. As we explore the world of nutrition, we will learn about the ingredients that drive excellent energy production and how to prepare balanced meals for long-term vitality.

Building Blocks of Vitality: Nutrients that Fuel Good Energy Production

Understanding the influence of diet on cellular energy begins with identifying the necessary nutrients that serve as the foundation of vitality. These nutrients each perform a unique function in powering the sophisticated machinery within our cells, ensuring that energy is produced consistently.

1. Carbohydrates: A Quick Energy Igniter

Carbohydrates, frequently referred to as the body's primary fuel source, act like high-octane gasoline, igniting the energy-producing process. These are present in foods such as grains, fruits, and vegetables. When carbs are ingested, they are converted into glucose, a simple sugar that is our cells' principal energy currency. Carbohydrates are like the fast-burning logs in the cellular hearth, delivering a rapid surge of energy to meet urgent requirements.

2. Proteins: The Cellular Architects and Repair Team

Proteins, which are commonly connected with muscle growth, serve an important function in cellular energy generation. These are the architects and repair technicians for our cellular constructions. Amino acids, the building blocks of proteins, play important roles in a variety of metabolic processes. They help to produce enzymes, which are necessary for nutrition breakdown and energy production. In our power plant example, proteins represent the skilled personnel who maintain and build various components of the energy producing facility.

3. Fats: Sustained Energy Reservoirs

Contrary to popular belief, fats are not the villains, but rather the sustained energy stores in our bodies. Healthy fats like avocados, almonds, and olive oil provide a long-lasting energy source. Fats are broken down into fatty acids, which enter energy production pathways, resulting in a gradual and consistent release of energy. Imagine lipids as slow-burning logs that provide a consistent and dependable supply of heat in our cellular fireplace.

4. Vitamins and Minerals: Micronutrient Support Team

Vitamins and minerals serve as the support team for the cellular power plant, maintaining its proper operation. These micronutrients function as cofactors and coenzymes, enabling a variety of metabolic pathways. B-vitamins, for example, play an important part in the digestion of carbs, proteins, and lipids, whereas minerals such as iron are required for enzymes involved in energy synthesis. Consider vitamins and minerals to be the maintenance team that maintains the power plant running smoothly and efficiently.

5. Hydration is the essential lubricant

Water, though sometimes forgotten, is the necessary lubricant that keeps the cellular machinery functioning properly. It acts as a medium for chemical processes that result in energy generation. Dehydration can cause slow metabolism and low energy production. Consider water to be the coolant that keeps the cellular power plant from overheating and maximizes energy generating efficiency.

Understanding these nutrient functions is critical for making educated choices about our daily nutritional intake. Just as a well-planned combination of diverse fuel sources keeps a power plant working smoothly, including a range of nutrients into our meals guarantees that our cellular power plant runs at its peak.

Creating Balanced Meals for Long-Term Vitality: The Art of Culinary Harmony

Now that we've learned about the importance of various nutrients, let's look at how to prepare balanced meals. Balancing carbs, proteins, lipids, vitamins, minerals, and water in our daily diet is similar to creating a symphony in which each component performs a distinct function, adding to the overall harmony of our nutritional intake.

1. The Plate Method: A Visual Guide to Balance

The plate technique is a simple and effective strategy to ensure that our meals have a balanced distribution of nutrients. Imagine splitting your dish into halves.

- **Half the Plate for Vegetables and Fruits:** These include critical vitamins, minerals, and fiber.
- **One-Quarter Protein:** Consume lean meats, chicken, fish, beans, or tofu for amino acids.
- **One-Quarter for Whole Grains or Healthy Carbohydrates:** Choose brown rice, quinoa, or whole-grain bread for long-lasting energy.
- **A Side of Healthy Fat:** To finish out your meal, add avocado, almonds, or olive oil.

This visual guide makes it easier to prepare balanced meals and ensures that your plate has a varied range of nutrients.

2. Snacking with Purpose: Micro-Meals for Sustainable Energy

In addition to main meals, snacks are essential for maintaining consistent energy levels throughout the day. Choose nutrient-dense snacks that contain carbs, protein, and healthy fats. For example, combine apple slices and nut butter, or Greek yogurt and berries. These micro-meals help to ensure that the cellular power plant has a constant supply of fuel, preventing energy crashes.

3. Hydration Habits: Quenching Cellular Thirsts

Hydration is sometimes overlooked, although it is an essential component of balanced diet. Aim to sip enough water throughout the day. Consider eating water-rich meals like fruits and vegetables to help you stay hydrated. Maintaining adequate fluid balance improves the efficiency of metabolic responses, resulting in optimal energy output.

4. Mindful Eating Enhances Nutrient Absorption

Beyond meal composition, how we eat effects nutritional absorption. Mindful eating is enjoying each mouthful, paying attention to hunger and fullness signals, and avoiding distractions. This method improves the body's capacity to take and absorb nutrients efficiently, enhancing the advantages of a well-balanced diet.

Conclusion: Fueling the Cellular Power Plant for Optimal Performance

In conclusion, Chapter 2 takes us on a tour through the influence of nutrition on cellular energy, comparing our bodies to complicated power plants powered by a range of nutrients. Understanding the functions of carbs, proteins, lipids, vitamins, minerals, and water gives us insight into how to create balanced meals that improve the performance of our cellular power plant.

As we continue our culinary adventure, the emphasis will be on the art of culinary harmony rather than restricted diets. Consider each meal to be a symphony, with diverse nutrients contributing to a harmonic balance of long-lasting vitality. The plate approach, mindful eating, and strategic snacking become our instruments for creating this nutritional symphony, ensuring that our cellular power plant runs at optimum efficiency and promotes long-term vitality and well-being. So, let us continue on this adventure, providing our bodies with the nutrition they require to survive and prosper.

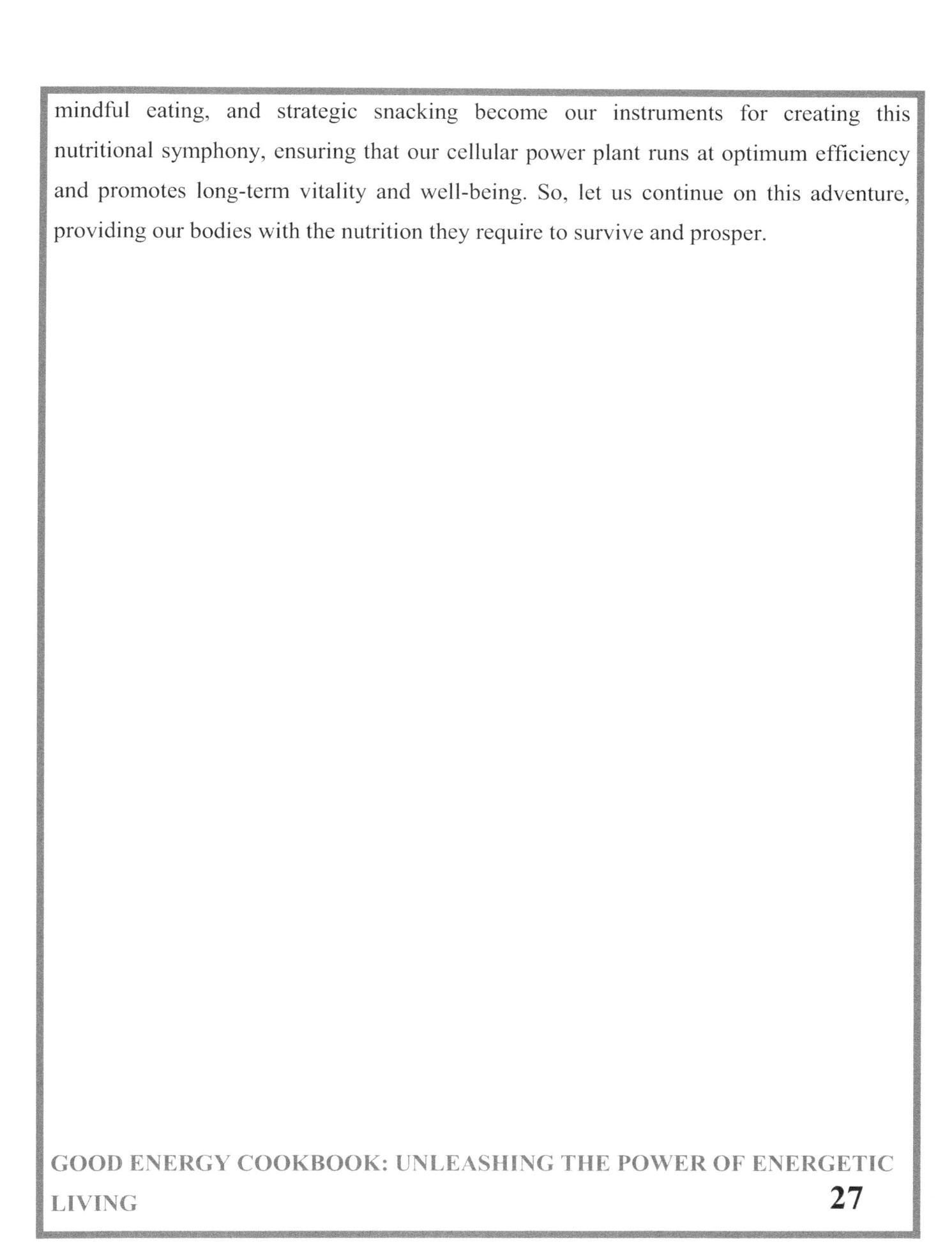

Chapter 3:

Recognizing the Signs of "Bad Energy" Foods and Navigating the Dietary Minefield

Beginning our investigation of metabolic health, Chapter 3 delves into the essential process of identifying "bad energy" meals. In this voyage, we will negotiate the culinary minefield, learning how some foods can upset the delicate balance of our metabolic systems. This chapter serves as a guide to recognizing these culprits and reveals ways for reducing dangerous food choices, allowing us to make educated decisions about our metabolic health.

Identifying Foods That Disrupt Metabolic Health: Unmasking the Causes

In the enormous array of dietary options, not all products are beneficial to our metabolic health. Some meals, frequently camouflaged as innocent perpetrators, can affect the proper functioning of our cellular power plant. Recognizing "bad energy" foods is critical for avoiding metabolic problems.

1. Refined Sugars and Processed Foods: Sweet Saboteurs

Excessive intake of refined sugars and processed meals is one of the leading causes of metabolic health issues. These products, which are common in many modern diets, cause fast rises in blood sugar levels. This causes an excessive insulin response, which may develop in insulin resistance over time. Insulin resistance occurs when cells become less sensitive to insulin, preventing the effective absorption of glucose. This may pave the path for type 2 diabetes and other metabolic diseases. Identifying and limiting the use of sugary drinks, sweets, pastries, and processed foods is an important step toward minimizing these hazards.

2. Trans and saturated fats: The Fat Foes

Fats are not all created equal, and some might be harmful to metabolic health. Trans fats, which are often present in industrially processed foods and some margarines, are especially infamous. They not only elevate LDL ("bad") cholesterol but also reduce HDL ("good") cholesterol, which contributes to cardiovascular disease. Saturated fats, which are commonly found in fatty cuts of meat and processed meals, can also cause inflammation and disrupt cellular function. Identifying and reducing the consumption of foods high in trans fats and saturated fats is critical for maintaining metabolic health.

3. High Alcohol Consumption: A Metabolic Disruptor

While moderate alcohol use may offer health advantages, excessive alcohol consumption can stress the liver, which is an important role in metabolic processes. The liver metabolizes alcohol, and prolonged alcohol intake can cause fatty liver disease and disturb complex metabolic processes. To protect metabolic health, recognize the indicators of excessive alcohol intake and establish mindful drinking practices.

4. Highly and ultra-processed foods: the convenience trap

Modern lives frequently cause us to consume highly processed and ultra-processed meals for convenience. These products, however, are frequently loaded with chemical additives, preservatives, and excessive quantities of salt and sugar. Regular intake can lead to inflammation, insulin resistance, and impaired metabolic function. Identifying and limiting your consumption of these convenience meals is critical for preserving the delicate balance of our metabolic processes.

Understanding these typical causes enables us to make more educated dietary selections, avoiding "bad energy" meals that may jeopardize our metabolic health.

Strategies for Minimizing Harmful Dietary Choices: A Roadmap to Healthier Eating Habits

Recognizing the indications of "bad energy" meals is only the first step; applying techniques to reduce their influence is the key to promoting long-term metabolic health. Here, we provide a road map for healthy eating habits, advising people on how to navigate the food minefield and make decisions that promote optimal metabolic function.

1. Reading Food Labels: Decoding Information

Learning to read food labels is one of the most effective ways for reducing unhealthy dietary choices. The ingredient list and nutritional information are useful for understanding a product's makeup. Look for hidden sugars, trans fats, and high salt levels. Choosing complete, minimally processed meals and goods with transparent ingredient labels enables people to make decisions that are beneficial to their metabolic health.

2. Prioritizing Whole Foods as Nutrient Powerhouses

Whole foods, in their original, unprocessed form, are nutritional powerhouses that promote metabolic health. These include fruits, vegetables, entire grains, lean proteins, and healthy fats. Prioritizing whole foods guarantees a varied diet of important nutrients while avoiding the chemicals and preservatives found in processed alternatives. Fill your plate with a variety of bright fruits and vegetables to provide a healthy amount of vitamins, minerals, and antioxidants.

3. Cooking at Home: Gaining Control Over Ingredients

Cooking at home allows us unequaled control over the ingredients utilized in meals. This not only improves flavor, but also enables people to make informed decisions regarding the quality of their food. Experimenting with herbs, spices, and cooking methods may turn whole foods into tasty and gratifying meals, making the transition to better eating more fun and sustainable.

4. Minimizing Added Sugars: A Sweet Victory for Metabolic Health

Added sugars, which are frequently found in unexpected areas, can play a significant role in metabolic disturbances. Limiting your intake of sugary beverages, candy, and processed foods is critical. Using natural sweeteners like honey or maple syrup in moderation can deliver a sweet triumph for metabolic health without sacrificing flavor.

5. Managing Alcohol Consumption: Mindful Sipping for Balance

For individuals who prefer alcoholic beverages, moderation is essential. Establishing mindful drinking practices, such as sipping gently, switching to water, and establishing boundaries, might help offset the possible detrimental consequences of excessive alcohol use on metabolic health.

6. Meal Planning and Prep: A Proactive Approach

Meal planning and preparing are effective strategies for maintaining healthy eating habits. Individuals who plan their meals ahead of time might make more deliberate decisions, resulting in a better nutritional balance. Preparing ingredients and meals in batches saves time and decreases dependency on prepackaged convenience foods. This proactive strategy establishes the foundation for regular and beneficial eating habits.

Conclusion: Navigating to Metabolic Resilience

As we finish Chapter 3, identifying the signals of "bad energy" meals becomes an important part of our road to metabolic resilience. Individuals may take control of their diet by identifying offenders such as refined carbohydrates, trans fats, excessive alcohol consumption, and highly processed foods.

Implementing techniques to reduce dangerous food choices creates a road map for improved eating habits. From reading food labels to emphasizing whole foods, cooking at home, and limiting alcohol consumption, these tactics help people navigate the nutritional maze with confidence.

As we progress in our search for metabolic well-being, these insights and methods become important guides, directing us toward a lifestyle that not only promotes optimal energy production but also promotes overall health and vitality. With each educated decision, we set the groundwork for a robust and harmonious metabolic orchestra, in which the foods we eat play an important part in creating a symphony of well-being. So, let us continue our trip with information and practices that will guide us to metabolic resilience and long-term health.

Chapter 4:

Monitoring Metabolic Health Through Diet—The Power of Biomarkers

In our continuous quest for optimal metabolic health, Chapter 4 focuses on a proactive approach: monitoring metabolic health through nutrition. This chapter investigates the use of biomarkers as powerful indicators for assessing our nutritional health, tracking progress, and making informed dietary changes. Consider biomarkers to be the dashboard of your metabolic engine, delivering real-time information on how well your body processes and uses the fuel you supply through your food.

Use Biomarkers to Assess Nutritional Status: Decoding the Body's Messages

Biomarkers are quantitative indicators found in our bodies that represent many elements of our health and wellness. When it comes to metabolic health, biomarkers are essential tools for understanding how our food choices affect our internal processes. Let's look at several significant indicators and what they say about our nutritional status:

1. Blood Glucose Levels: The Sugar Balance Indicator

Blood glucose levels are an important indicator, providing information about how well your body processes carbs. Elevated blood glucose levels, particularly after meals, may suggest insulin resistance. Monitoring these levels allows you to understand how different foods affect your blood sugar and helps you make changes to maintain consistent energy levels throughout the day.

2. Cholesterol Levels: The Lipid Profile for Cardiovascular Health

Cholesterol levels, including LDL ("bad") and HDL ("good") cholesterol, reflect your lipid profile. Elevated LDL levels may indicate an imbalance in fat metabolism, raising the risk of cardiovascular disease. Monitoring cholesterol levels enables proactive dietary changes, such as lowering saturated and trans fats, to improve cardiovascular health.

3. Inflammation Markers: Determining Internal Stress Levels

Inflammation indicators, such as C-reactive protein (CRP), indicate the amount of inflammation in the body. Chronic inflammation is linked to a variety of health concerns, including metabolic diseases. Monitoring inflammation indicators allows people to discover potential triggers in their diet and make changes to minimize inflammatory reactions.

4. Nutrient Levels: Assessing Micronutrient Status

Regular blood testing can determine the amounts of vital nutrients such as vitamin D, B12, iron, and others. Deficiencies in these micronutrients can have an influence on metabolism and general health. Monitoring vitamin levels might help you change your diet or consider taking supplements to treat particular deficits.

5. Hemoglobin A1c, the Long-Term Blood Sugar Gauge

Hemoglobin A1c is a measurement that shows the average blood sugar levels over the previous several months. This gives a more complete picture of blood sugar management and helps spot trends that may necessitate dietary changes. It is especially beneficial for people who have diabetes or are at risk of developing it.

Tracking Progress and Making Informed Dietary Changes: A Personalized Approach

Now that we understand the importance of these biomarkers, the next step is to use them to assess development and make educated dietary decisions. It's vital to remember that everyone is different, and there is no one-size-fits-all strategy to food. A customized and iterative strategy enables fine-tuning food choices based on individual reactions and changing health goals.

1. Regular Monitoring: Creating a Baseline
Begin by establishing a baseline through frequent monitoring of important biomarkers. Depending on the biomarkers being tracked, this might include routine blood tests, continuous glucose monitoring, or other approaches. Setting a baseline enables you to better understand your body's natural changes and detect any deviations that may indicate the need for modification.

2. Food Diary: Connect the Dots

Keeping a food diary can be an effective way to correlate dietary decisions with biomarker changes. Keep a record of everything you eat, when you consume it, and how you feel afterwards. This approach aids in the identification of patterns and connections between certain diets and biomarker levels. For example, you may find that particular meals cause raised blood sugar levels or inflammation.

3. Experimentation: Managing Dietary Changes

Experiment with dietary adjustments based on the data collected from biomarkers and your food diary. This might include altering macronutrient ratios, investigating the effect of certain foods on blood sugar, or adding more nutrient-dense alternatives. Small, gradual modifications allow you to monitor your body's response and make adjustments based on real-time input.

4. Expert Guidance for Consultants in Healthcare

Consult with healthcare specialists, such as dietitians and nutritionists, to understand biomarker data and obtain individualized counsel. These specialists can help you understand the consequences of biomarker patterns, make evidence-based suggestions, and work with you to develop a long-term and effective dietary plan.

5. Listening to Your Body: Tune into Signals

Beyond biomarkers, it is critical to listen to your body's cues. Pay attention to hunger and fullness signals, energy levels, and how different meals make you feel. This intuitive approach, along with biomarker insights, leads to a comprehensive knowledge of your body's specific demands.

Conclusion: Empowering with Knowledge and Action

Finally, monitoring metabolic health through nutrition allows people to take an active role in their own health. Biomarkers are useful tools, providing real-time insights into how dietary choices affect internal processes. Individuals may adapt their diet to promote optimal metabolic function by analyzing and measuring blood glucose levels, cholesterol levels, inflammatory indicators, nutrition levels, and hemoglobin A1c.

Tracking progress and making smart dietary changes becomes a customized journey aided by data and individual reactions. The combination of frequent monitoring, dietary diaries, experimentation, professional advice, and intuitive listening results in a complete approach to metabolic health.

As we continue our pursuit for metabolic well-being, equipped with information and the capacity to analyze biomarker data, we lay the groundwork for a healthier and more robust future. This proactive and tailored approach turns the quest for optimal metabolic health into an empowering and informative experience. So, let us continue our investigation, relying on biomarkers to guide us along the route to long-term health and vitality.

Chapter 5:

Creating a Good Energy Meal Plan--A Four-Week Blueprint for Optimal Health

As we enter Chapter 5, the focus shifts to creating a Good Energy Meal Plan, a complete four-week plan designed to fuel optimal health. This chapter is about more than simply what we eat; it is about converting our dietary habits into a sustainable lifestyle that promotes well-being. We'll look at the art of creating a meal plan that includes diversity and balance, setting the groundwork for long-term success on the path to excellent energy.

Developing a Four-Week Meal Plan for Optimal Health: The Architecture of Well-Being

Developing a meal plan for maximum health entails more than simply deciding what to eat for breakfast, lunch, and supper. It is about knowing the body's nutritional demands, combining a variety of food sources, and tailoring meals to specific health objectives. Let's break down the process into manageable stages for creating a four-week food plan that promotes healthy energy.

1. Assessing Nutritional Needs: A Personal Approach

Begin by determining your nutritional requirements based on age, gender, activity level, and health objectives. This stage establishes the groundwork for a tailored food plan that suits your individual needs. Consider speaking with a healthcare expert or a qualified dietician to guarantee accurate evaluations and personalized advice.

2. Understanding Macronutrient Ratios: The Building Blocks of Energy.

Macronutrients, which include carbs, proteins, and lipids, serve as the foundation for energy production. Understanding the best ratios for your specific needs is critical. For example, someone who engages in frequent physical activity may require a larger proportion of carbs to maintain energy levels, but those who focus on muscle growth may require a higher protein consumption. Balancing these macronutrients is essential for sustaining energy throughout the day.

3. Incorporating Micronutrients: A Nutrient Symphony

Micronutrients, such as vitamins and minerals, are necessary for a variety of biological activities. A well-balanced meal plan should include a mix of fruits and vegetables, whole grains, lean meats, and healthy fats to guarantee an adequate amount of micronutrients. Each food category adds a distinct collection of vitamins and minerals, resulting in a nutritional symphony that promotes general health.

4. Meal Timing and Frequency: Providing Consistent Nutrition for the Body

The timing and frequency of meals affects energy levels, metabolism, and general well-being. To manage blood sugar levels and avoid energy dumps, plan meals on a constant schedule. Consider the benefits of spacing your meals throughout the day, including snacks as needed, to maintain a consistent supply of nutrients and avoid overeating during main meals.

5. Hydration: the Overlooked Elixir

Water is often forgotten when preparing meals, despite its importance in supporting metabolic functions and general health. Drink plenty of water throughout the day and eat water-rich meals like fruits and vegetables. Hydration improves digestion, food absorption, and energy levels.

A Sample Four-Week Meal Plan that Balances Nutrition and Variety

Let's put these concepts into practice by creating an example four-week food plan. This plan is intended to give ideas and a starting point for creating a sustainable and healthy routine. Remember to customize the plan depending on personal tastes, dietary constraints, and special health objectives.

Week 1: Breakfast, Lunch, Dinner and Snacks

Day 1:
 - Breakfast: Oatmeal with berries and nuts
- Lunch: Grilled chicken salad with mixed greens, cherry tomatoes, cucumbers, and vinaigrette

- Dinner: Baked salmon with quinoa and steamed broccoli
- Snacks: Greek yogurt with honey and almonds

Day 15:
- Breakfast: Whole-grain toast with avocado and poached eggs
- Lunch: Lentil soup with mixed vegetables
- Dinner: Stir-fried tofu with brown rice and colorful bell peppers
- Snack: Sliced apple with peanut butter

Week 2:
- Day 1: Same as Week 1
- Day 15 Introduce a new breakfast alternative by blending spinach, banana, Greek yogurt, and a scoop of protein powder.

Week 3:
- Day 1: Try a breakfast dish with quinoa, berries, and Greek yogurt.
- Day 15: Include a meal of grilled shrimp skewers with quinoa and roasted Brussels sprouts.

Week 4:
- Day 1: Prepare a breakfast frittata with eggs, spinach, tomatoes, and feta cheese.
- Day 15:. Try a vegetarian meal of chickpea and vegetable curry served with brown rice.

Adding Variety and Balance for Long-Term Success: The Key to Culinary Harmony

As we create our four-week meal plan, the emphasis on diversity and balance becomes critical to long-term success. Variety not only makes meals more pleasurable, but it also provides a varied range of nutrients. Balancing different dietary categories gives the body the critical nutrients it requires for optimal operation.

1. Explore Culinary Diversity: A Feast for the Senses.

Incorporate a variety of fruits, vegetables, whole grains, lean meats, and healthy fats into your food plan. Use various cooking methods, spices, and herbs to enhance the flavor and attractiveness of your food. Culinary diversity not only makes meals more fascinating, but it also broadens the range of nutrients your body absorbs.

2. Mindful Eating: Enjoying Every Bite

Include mindful eating habits in your meal plan. Take time to taste each meal, appreciate the flavors, and pay attention to your body's hunger and fullness signs. Mindful eating improves the entire dining experience and fosters a better connection with food.

3. Adaptability and Flexibility: A Dynamic Approach

Recognize that life is always changing, therefore your food plan should be adjustable. Be willing to test new recipes, change portion proportions, and accommodate special events. This flexibility guarantees that your food plan is both practical and sustainable in the long run.

4. Portion Control: Quality vs Quantity

While diversity is important, so is portion management. To avoid overeating, keep your portion proportions in check. Prioritize nutrient-dense foods that include vital vitamins, minerals, and macronutrients.

5. Social and Cultural Influences: Nourish the Soul

Consider the social and cultural components of your eating plan. Sharing meals with family and friends, as well as trying new foods from other cultures, may be meaningful experiences. Nourishing not just the body but also the psyche promotes a holistic approach to well-being.

Conclusion: A Culinary Symphony for Long-Term Health

Finally, developing a Good Energy Meal Plan is similar to creating a culinary symphony - a harmonic combination of nutrients, diversity, and balance. A four-week plan requires analyzing dietary needs, establishing macronutrient ratios, and combining micronutrients to create a nutrient symphony that promotes optimal health.

Our sample four-week meal plan serves as a starting point, stressing variety and adaptability. Balancing nutrition with gastronomic diversity, mindful eating, flexibility, portion management, and cultural influences results in a dynamic approach to meal planning. This culinary symphony is not a rigorous set of rules,

Flexible guidance that adapts to individual preferences and health goals.

As we begin on the road of long-term well-being, let us approach our meal planning with originality, curiosity, and fun. With each well-balanced and healthy meal, we contribute to the symphony of long-term health, cultivating positive energy that vibrates throughout our bodies. So, let us continue our culinary journey, relishing the tastes of a well-crafted meal plan that nourishes not just our bodies but also our total sense of vigor and joy.

Chapter 6:

Principles of Good Energy Eating—Unraveling Dietary Philosophies for Lifelong Health

In Chapter 6, we will explore the Principles of Good Energy Eating. This chapter serves as a guide to dismantling popular dietary beliefs and fallacies, allowing people to make educated decisions that contribute to lifetime health. Let us untangle the intricacies of food, comprehend the science behind diverse dietary methods, and put sustainable food ideas into action that will last.

Understanding Dietary Philosophies and Myths: Navigating the Food Maze

The realm of nutrition is sometimes fraught with contradicting advice, trends, and fallacies. From fad diets promising fast solutions to sensationalized claims about particular foods, navigating the food maze may be difficult. Let's look at some prevalent dietary philosophies and misconceptions to separate the science from the hype.

1. Low-Fat vs. Low-Carb Dilemma: The Macronutrient Battle

In the debate over low-fat and low-carb diets, it is critical to recognize that both macronutrients play important functions in our diet. Vilifying one above the other simplifies our body's intricate interaction with lipids and carbs. Rather of going to extremes, adopt a balanced diet rich in healthy fats and complex carbs derived from whole foods.

2. Myth about "Magic" Foods: No Panacea Exists

The concept of "magic" meals with amazing health effects is a pervasive misconception. While many meals are high in nutrients and promote well-being, no single diet can cure all illnesses or ensure eternal health. Instead of looking for a miracle cure, prioritize a broad, nutrient-dense diet.

3. Detox Diets: Identifying Facts from Fiction

Detox diets frequently promise to rid the body of toxins and encourage quick weight reduction. However, the body has built-in detoxification mechanisms, which are primarily controlled by the liver and kidneys. Extreme detox regimens may cause nutritional deficits and are often unsustainable. Instead, eat a well-balanced diet rich in nutritious foods to help your body's natural detoxification processes.

4. The Gluten-Free Craze: Navigating Sensitivities

The gluten-free trend has grown in popularity, with some viewing gluten as a health risk. While people with gluten sensitivities or celiac disease must avoid gluten, going gluten-free may not provide any additional health benefits in the general population. It is critical to distinguish between medical necessity and dietary trends when making food choices.

5. Superfood Hype: The Truth About Nutrient-Rich Foods

The term "superfood" is frequently used to describe foods that are said to provide extraordinary health benefits. While nutrient-dense foods such as berries, leafy greens, and nuts contain a variety of vitamins, minerals, and antioxidants, no single superfood can transform health on its own. Accept a wide range of nutrient-dense foods to ensure a balanced and comprehensive nutritional intake.

A Comprehensive Approach to Implementing Sustainable Food Principles for Long-Term Health

After debunking myths and navigating dietary philosophies, the next step is to put sustainable food principles into action to promote long-term health. These principles go beyond quick fixes and restrictive diets, emphasizing a holistic approach to nutrition.

1. Whole Food Focus: Accepting Nutrient Density

Prioritizing whole, nutrient-dense foods is essential for good energy eating. Whole foods in their natural state contain a wide range of vitamins, minerals, fiber, and other essential nutrients. These foods provide comprehensive nutrition to the body, promoting optimal metabolic function and overall health.

- **Practical Tip:** Fill your plate with a variety of colorful fruits and vegetables, whole grains, lean proteins, and healthy fats. This approach ensures a broad spectrum of nutrients that contribute to sustained energy and vitality.

2. Moderation and Balance: Avoiding Extremes

The principle of moderation and balance acknowledges the importance of enjoying a variety of foods without deprivation or excess. It's about finding equilibrium and savoring the pleasures of food. Restrictive diets often lead to frustration and are challenging to maintain in the long run. Instead, embrace a balanced approach that allows for flexibility and enjoyment.

- **Practical Tip:** Indulge in your favorite treats occasionally, but ensure that the majority of your meals are balanced and nourishing. This balance fosters a positive relationship with food and supports sustainable dietary habits.

3. Individualized Nutrition: Recognizing Bioindividuality

Each person is unique, and there is no one-size-fits-all approach to nutrition. Bioindividuality recognizes that individuals have different dietary needs based on factors like genetics, lifestyle, and health goals. Tailoring your food choices to your individual requirements ensures a more personalized and effective approach to good energy eating.

- **Practical Tip:** Listen to your body's signals, pay attention to how different foods make you feel, and adapt your diet based on your unique preferences and needs.

4. Mindful Eating: Enhancing the Dining Experience

Mindful eating is a practice that encourages full awareness and presence during meals. It involves savoring each bite, paying attention to hunger and fullness cues, and avoiding distractions. This approach fosters a deeper connection with food, enhances digestion, and promotes a healthier relationship with eating.

- **Practical Tip:** Turn off electronic devices, savor the flavors of your meals, and listen to your body's signals. Mindful eating transforms meals into more than just a physical necessity; it becomes a mindful and enjoyable experience.

5. Seasonal and Local Choices: Supporting Sustainability

Choosing seasonal and local foods not only benefits the environment but also enhances the nutritional quality of your meals. Seasonal produce is often fresher and more nutrient-dense, while supporting local farmers contributes to sustainable agriculture practices.

- **Practical Tip:** Explore local farmers' markets, embrace seasonal produce, and incorporate a variety of fruits and vegetables that align with the changing seasons.

Conclusion: Nourishing a Lifetime of Good Energy

In conclusion, the Principles of Good Energy Eating provide a roadmap for lifelong health by dispelling dietary myths and embracing sustainable food principles. The journey involves recognizing the nuances of different dietary philosophies, debunking myths, and adopting an approach that focuses on whole foods, balance, individualized nutrition, mindful eating, and sustainability.

As we incorporate these principles into our daily lives, we nourish not only our bodies but also

our overall sense of well-being. Good energy eating becomes a holistic practice that extends beyond the dinner plate, influencing our energy levels, mood, and vitality. So, let's continue this journey with curiosity and openness, savoring the flavors of a well-balanced and sustainable approach to nutrition, and nurturing a lifetime of good energy.

Chapter 7

Improving Sleep and Circadian Rhythm for Better Metabolism: Unlocking the Power of Rest

In Chapter 7, we will look at the often-overlooked cornerstones of health: sleep and circadian rhythm. The fundamental link between excellent sleep, a well-regulated circadian rhythm, and healthy metabolism serves as the foundation of our investigation. We will investigate the complex link between sleep and energy balance, diving into the science, and then arm ourselves with practical ways to improve sleep quality and rhythm for general well-being.

Understanding the Relationship between Sleep and Energy Balance: The Sleep-Metabolism Nexus

Sleep is more than just a condition of rest; it is a dynamic and necessary process that affects almost every element of our well-being. The complicated dance between sleep and metabolism is critical for maintaining energy balance, impacting weight control, hormone modulation, and general well-being.

1. Hormonal Harmony: Leptin, Ghrelin, and Insulin

Sleep has a significant impact on hormonal control, notably for hormones such as leptin, ghrelin, and insulin. Leptin, the hormone that signals fullness, diminishes with little sleep, resulting in increased appetite. On the other hand, ghrelin, the hormone that drives appetite, increases. This hormonal imbalance can lead to overeating and weight gain.

Furthermore, poor sleep can cause insulin resistance, affecting blood sugar levels and raising the risk of type 2 diabetes.

2. Cortisol Control and Stress Hormone Dynamics

Cortisol, a hormone linked with stress, has a natural circadian cycle. Disruptions in sleep habits can disrupt this cycle, resulting in high cortisol levels at inappropriate periods. This hormone imbalance not only impacts energy metabolism, but it also leads to stress-related problems including anxiety and mood swings.

3. Energy Expenditure: The Restorative Power Of Sleep

Quality sleep is inextricably connected to energy consumption and the body's capacity to recuperate. During deep sleep, the body repairs and restores itself, which includes the release of growth hormone, muscle repair, and memory consolidation. These functions help to maintain overall metabolic health, which influences both physical and mental well-being.

Practical Strategies for Improving Sleep Quality and Rhythm: The Road to Relaxing Nights

Now that we understand the significance of the sleep-metabolism relationship, let's set out on a quest to improve sleep quality and control circadian rhythm. This initiative is built on practical ideas, which provide real actions for creating an atmosphere favorable to peaceful sleep.

1. Creating a Consistent Sleep Schedule: Harmonizing with Circadian Rhythms

Circadian rhythms are internal 24-hour cycles that control a variety of physiological functions, including sleep-wake patterns. Aligning our sleep cycle with these natural rhythms promotes better sleep quality. Aim for a constant bedtime and wake-up time, including on weekends, to help the body's internal clock.

 - **Practical Tip:** Establish a consistent bedtime and wake-up time to create a sleep habit that tells your body when it's time to relax and when it's time to wake up.

2. Developing a Sleep-Conducive Environment: The Sanctuary of Rest

Transform your bedroom into a slumber paradise. Keep the room dark, quiet, and chilly. Invest on soft bedding and a supportive mattress. To create the best sleeping environment, reduce noise and light interruptions and consider utilizing blackout curtains.

 - **Practical Tip** Dim the lights one hour before sleep to indicate to your body that it is time to relax. Remove electronic gadgets that generate blue light, as this sort of light might interfere with the generation of melatonin, a hormone required for sleep.

3. Reducing Stimulants and Electronic Device Use: Managing Sleep Disruptors

Caffeine, nicotine, and electronic gadgets can all interfere with falling asleep and getting a good night's sleep. Limit your stimulant consumption, particularly in the evening, and develop a pre-sleep regimen that excludes screen usage.

- **Practical Tip** Avoid coffee in the hours preceding up to bedtime, and consider setting up a technology-free zone at least 30 minutes before bed. Read a book or stretch gently to help you relax.

4. Regular Exercise: Energizing Days and Restful Nights

Regular physical exercise has a beneficial effect on sleep quality. Exercise stimulates endorphin release, decreases stress, and helps regulate circadian cycles. However, it is critical to timing exercise correctly; hard exercises near bedtime may have a stimulating impact.

- **Practical Tip** Incorporate physical activity into your regular routine, but try to do more strenuous workouts early in the day. Gentle activities, such as yoga or strolling in the evening, might help you relax.

5. Mindfulness and Relaxation Techniques to Calm the Mind and Body

Incorporating mindfulness and relaxation practices into your pre-sleep routine helps alert your body that it's time to rest. Deep breathing, meditation, and gradual muscle relaxation can all help to calm the mind and establish a sleep-inducing state.

- **Practical Tip:** Spend a few minutes before bedtime doing mindfulness exercises. This might involve deep breathing exercises, meditation programs, or moderate stretches to relieve tension.

6. Strategic Exposure to Light: Unlocking the Power of Natural Light

Exposure to natural light during the day helps to regulate circadian rhythms and supports the body's internal clock. Spend time outside during the daytime hours, particularly in the morning. Reduce your exposure to intense artificial light in the evening to inform your body that it is time to prepare for sleep.

- **Practical Tip** During the day, aim to spend at least 30 minutes outside in natural light. Dim the lights and lower screen brightness in the evening to signify the start of the night.

7. Balanced Fluid Intake: Hydrating Wisely

While being hydrated is important for general health, drinking too much fluid prior to bedtime might cause disturbed nightly awakenings. Stay hydrated throughout the day, and consider limiting fluid consumption in the hours.

Leading up to nighttime.

- **Practical Tip:** Hydrate sufficiently during the day and reduce fluid consumption in the evening. This reduces the probability of waking up throughout the night for potty breaks.

Conclusion: A Symphony of Sleep and Metabolism

In conclusion, Chapter 7 has revealed the complex relationship between sleep, circadian rhythm, and metabolism. Understanding the influence of sleep on hormone control, energy expenditure, and general well-being highlights the significance of getting enough rest for a balanced and healthy existence.

Armed with realistic solutions, we set out to improve sleep quality and control circadian rhythm. This transforming attempt is built on establishing a consistent sleep schedule, building a sleep-conducive atmosphere, minimizing stimulants, exercising regularly, adding mindfulness techniques, selective light exposure, and regulating fluid intake.

As we embrace the concepts of sleep hygiene and circadian rhythm alignment, we help to create a health symphony that echoes throughout our bodies. The harmonious interaction of sleep and metabolism becomes a pillar of total health, promoting energy balance, hormonal equilibrium, and a robust life. So, let us continue this journey by committing to peaceful nights, fostering the critical link between sleep and metabolic health, and creating a symphony of renewal and energy.

Chapter 8

Integrating Movement and Exercise for Metabolic Health

The Dance of Daily Activity and Purposeful Exercise

In Chapter 8, we delve into the dynamic world of movement and exercise, investigating how these factors work together to improve metabolic health. This chapter seeks to clarify the notions of physical activity and exercise, emphasizing the need of incorporating both daily motions and planned exercises into our lives. Let's look at the necessity of including everyday activities to boost physical activity and how to create a balanced workout program that helps to overall wellbeing.

Embracing Everyday Activities to Increase Physical Activity: The Power of Movement

Physical exercise is not limited to planned workouts; it includes all of our daily motions. These seemingly basic tasks, such as ascending the stairs or walking the dog, have a substantial impact on our overall physical health. Recognizing and accepting the importance of everyday motions paves the way for a comprehensive approach to metabolic health.

1. Non-Exercise Activity Thermogenesis (NEAT): Small Steps, Big Impact.

Non-exercise activity. Thermogenesis (NEAT) is the energy expended during non-exercise activities like walking, standing, or fidgeting. While these behaviors may appear little, the cumulative impact can be significant. NEAT makes up a considerable amount of our daily energy expenditure, which influences metabolic health and weight control.

- Practical Tip:

Look for ways to boost NEAT throughout the day. Take short breaks to stand, walk, or stretch, and consider adding movement into normal chores, such as using a standing desk or using the stairs rather than the elevator.

2. Everyday Movement and Metabolism: A symbiotic relationship

Everyday activity is essential for maintaining metabolic health. Regular low-intensity exercises help to improve insulin sensitivity, blood sugar management, and cardiovascular performance. These little motions not only burn calories, but also improve the general efficiency of our metabolic processes.

- Practical Tip:

Find delight in ordinary tasks that require mobility. Gardening, dancing, and playing with children are all hobbies that not only improve metabolic health but also bring fun to our everyday routines.

3. Walking as a Fundamental Exercise: Steps to Metabolic Wellness

Walking, a simple and accessible type of exercise, has significant advantages for metabolic health. It increases calorie expenditure while also improving cardiovascular fitness, mood, and joint health. Walking is a fantastic beginning point for individuals who want to become more physically active.

- Practical Tip

Incorporate walking into your daily routine by walking small distances instead of driving, taking a stroll after meals, or visiting nearby nature trails. Gradually raise your daily step count to gain the metabolic advantages of this easy yet effective workout.

4. Posture and Movement Awareness: Aligning for Health

Posture and body alignment are essential parts of everyday activity that are often overlooked. Maintaining excellent posture and being mindful of our movements can help avoid musculoskeletal problems and improve overall health. Simple modifications, such as sitting with a straight back or lifting items with good form, help to create the harmonic dance of daily movement.

- Practical Tip

Pay attention to your posture when sitting at a desk or waiting in line. Make deliberate attempts to keep your spine neutral, activate your core muscles, and move with purpose.

Creating a Balanced Exercise Routine for Overall Health: Purposeful Movement

While everyday activities are the cornerstone of physical activity, purposeful exercise adds an organized and intentional component to our movement repertoire. Building a balanced exercise regimen entails integrating a variety of workouts that target different parts of fitness while improving overall wellbeing and metabolic health.

1. Cardiovascular Exercise: Fueling the Heart and Metabolism

Cardiovascular workouts, often called aerobic exercises, increase heart rate and respiration. This category covers running, cycling, swimming, and dancing. Cardiovascular exercise promotes cardiovascular health, increases circulation, and aids in weight loss by burning calories.

- Practical Tip:

To make exercise more fun, choose cardiovascular activities that interest you. Whether it's a dancing class, a brisk walk, or a bike ride, pick an activity that gets your heart rate up while still fitting into your schedule.

2. Strength Training for Metabolic Resilience

Strength training is working against resistance to increase muscle strength and endurance. Contrary to popular belief, strength training benefits everyone, not just bodybuilders. Increased muscle mass improves metabolism, insulin sensitivity, and overall metabolic resistance.

- Practical Tip

Incorporate strength training workouts into your program at least twice or three times each week. This might include bodyweight workouts, weighted resistance training, or strength and flexibility-focused activities such as yoga.

3. Flexibility and Mobility: Fluid Motion

Flexibility and mobility exercises improve the general functionality of the body. Stretching and yoga are two practices that enhance range of motion, lower the risk of injury, and generate a sense of comfort in movement. Flexibility and mobility exercises supplement other types of exercise, resulting in a well-rounded approach to health.

- Practical Tip:

Make time for stretching exercises or attend yoga classes on a regular basis. These workouts not only improve flexibility but also promote calm and awareness.

4. High-Intensity Interval Training (HIIT): Efficiency in Movement

High-intensity interval training consists of brief
Bursts of vigorous exercise are followed by short intervals of rest or lower-intensity activity. HIIT is well-known for its ability to burn calories quickly, improve cardiovascular fitness, and promote metabolic adaptations. These routines are time-efficient and adaptable to different fitness levels.

- Practical Tip:

Try introducing HIIT exercises into your program, beginning with shorter periods and progressively increasing intensity. Consult with a fitness specialist to determine whether HIIT is appropriate for your fitness level and health situation.

5. Mind-Body Practices: Balancing Physical and Mental Health

Mind-body practices, such as tai chi and qigong, highlight the link between physical movement and mental well-being. These techniques help to induce relaxation, reduce tension, and maintain a feeling of equilibrium. Integrating mind-body activities into your daily routine promotes a comprehensive approach to wellness.

- Practical Tip:

Investigate mind-body techniques that appeal to you. Attend a tai chi class, practice mindful movement, or add deep breathing techniques into your daily routine to get the advantages of both physical and emotional well-being.

Creating Your Personal Movement Symphony: A Lifelong Journey.

Building a balanced exercise program and using everyday activities to improve physical activity is a lifetime process that changes with individual preferences, objectives, and health condition. It is not about following a strict set of rules, but about creating a movement symphony that offers joy, vigor, and long-term health.

1. Personalizing Your Movement Journey: Listen to Your Body.

Recognize that everyone's mobility requirements are unique. Listen to your body, pay attention to its signals, and customize your workout regimen to fit your tastes and physical condition. Personalizing your activity path ensures that it is both sustainable and fun.

- Practical Tip

Experiment with various workouts and activities to see what resonates with you. Find movement forms that fulfill you, whether it's dance, hiking, or martial arts.

2. Gradual Progression: A Path to Long-Term Success

Avoid the urge to start an aggressive fitness routine overnight. Gradual growth is critical for long-term success and injury avoidance. Begin with simple activities, gradually increasing the intensity and time as your fitness improves.

- Practical Tip:

Set achievable objectives and milestones for your fitness journey. Celebrate minor triumphs and be patient with yourself as you steadily increase endurance and strength.

3. Consistency Over Intensity: Building Habits for Life

Consistency is the foundation of every effective movement regimen. Concentrate on developing habits that value consistent physical activity over irregular, intensive sessions. Consistent physical activity, even in tiny doses, has long-term metabolic health advantages.

- Practical Tip:

Schedule time for physical activity. This might be as easy as going for a brief stroll during lunch breaks, including stretching into your daily routine, or doing a fast exercise before or after work.

4. Enjoyment as a Motivator: Making Movement a Pleasureful Experience

When activity is joyful, it becomes an integral part of daily life. Find things that make you happy, whether it's the companionship of group courses, the isolation of a nature walk, or the pleasure of meeting personal fitness goals.

- Practical Tip:

Experiment with several types of exercise until you discover something you truly love. Consider experimenting with different things on a regular basis to keep your routine interesting.

5. Social Connection via Movement: A Supportive Community

Participating in physical activity with others promotes a sense of community and support. Joining a sports team, taking group lessons, or going for a stroll with friends all improve motivation and pleasure of physical activity.

- Practical Tip:

Seek for opportunities to move with others. This might be taking a local fitness class, attending community events, or inviting others to join you in your favorite physical activities.

Conclusion: A Symphony of Movement for Metabolic Harmony

In conclusion, Chapter 8 has demonstrated the transforming effect of combining movement and exercise for metabolic health. This chapter highlights a comprehensive approach to movement, from embracing ordinary activities that promote increased physical activity to developing a balanced workout program.

Recognizing the importance of everyday motions and intentional workouts results in a symphony of movement that promotes general well-being. The rhythmic dance of walking, the strength-building crescendo of resistance training, and the soothing tones of flexibility exercises all contribute to the harmonic interplay of metabolic health.

As we begin our personal exercise adventure, let us approach it with curiosity, enthusiasm, and a dedication to long-term health. By incorporating activity into our everyday lives, we not only improve our metabolic health but also develop a lively and satisfying lifestyle. So, let the movement symphony begin - a lifetime quest for metabolic balance, vigor, and a healthier, more joyful existence.

Chapter 9

Exploring the Benefits of Temperature Exposure

Harnessing the Power of Cold and Heat for Metabolic Resilience

In Chapter 9, we start on an exciting investigation into the effects of temperature exposure on metabolic health. This chapter delves into the realms of cold and heat, revealing the surprising advantages that temperature fluctuations may have on our health. From increasing metabolic resilience to improving general well-being, we'll look at the science underpinning temperature exposure and detail safe and effective ways to incorporate these aspects into our daily lives.

Using Cold to Improve Metabolic Resilience: The Icy Path to Health

Cold exposure, which is frequently linked with chills and pain, has a surprising number of advantages for metabolic resilience. Understanding how our bodies respond to cold stimuli reveals the therapeutic benefits of embracing the chill.

1. Activation of Brown Adipose Tissue (BAT): The Metabolic Furnace

Brown adipose tissue (BAT) is a form of fat that has a distinct role in energy expenditure. Unlike white adipose tissue, which stores energy, BAT produces heat by burning calories.

Cold stimulates BAT, transforming it into a metabolic furnace that regulates body temperature and aids in calorie burning.

- Practical Tip

Incorporate brief cold exposures into your daily routine, such as having a cold shower or spending a few minutes in a chilly room. Gradually extend the duration as your body adjusts.

2. Increased Caloric Expenditure: Shivering as a Metabolic Exercise

Shivering, a natural response to cold, is more than just a source of discomfort; it's also a metabolic exercise. Shivering causes an increase in calorie expenditure as the body strives to create heat. This involuntary exercise can help with weight control and metabolic health.

- Practical Tip:

Enjoy the odd shiver-inducing event, whether it's a chilly stroll or being in a cold place. Dress correctly to ensure safety and progressively increase tolerance.

3. Improved Insulin Sensitivity with Cold as a Metabolic Reset

Cold exposure has been associated to enhanced insulin sensitivity, which is an important aspect in metabolic health. Increased insulin sensitivity indicates that cells respond more efficiently to insulin, allowing for more effective blood sugar regulation. This can help to lower the risk of type 2 diabetes and enhance overall metabolic function.

GOOD ENERGY COOKBOOK: UNLEASHING THE POWER OF ENERGETIC LIVING

- **Practical Tip** Experiment with cold exposure methods like ice baths and cold-water immersions. Begin with shorter periods and speak with a healthcare practitioner, especially if you have pre-existing health concerns.

4. Stress Resilience and Hormonal Balance: Cold as a Hormic Stressor

Cold exposure is a hormetic stressor, which means it causes a moderate stress reaction in the body, resulting in positive adaptations. This stress resistance goes beyond metabolic health, altering hormonal balance and increasing overall resilience.

- Practical Tip

Introduce cold exposure gradually, enabling your body to adjust. Start with less extreme versions, such as concluding your shower with a rush of cold water, then work your way up to more immersing experiences.

Safe and Effective Practices for Cold Exposure: Navigating the Chill.

While the benefits of cold exposure are clear, it is critical to adopt these activities cautiously and gradually. Sudden or extended exposure to severe cold can be dangerous, so following these guidelines responsibly provides a pleasurable and health-promoting experience.

1. Begin Gradually: Adjusting to the Cold

Cold exposure is most beneficial when used gradually. Begin with shorter, less intense sessions to allow your body to adjust. This progressive approach reduces the danger of unpleasant responses while increasing the body's potential to adjust positively.

- Practical Tip

If you're new to cold exposure, start with short cold showers or walks in chilly weather. As your body adjusts, you may progressively increase the time and intensity of your cold exposure.

2. Consider Individual Tolerance: Personalized Cold Practices

Individuals' tolerance for cold might vary. When adopting cold exposure strategies, it is important to consider age, health state, and individual sensitivity. Tailor your approach to your degree of comfort and any current health issues.

- Practical Tip:

Pay attention to how your body reacts to frigid temperatures. If you have any health issues or conditions, speak with a doctor before beginning more rigorous cold practices.

3. Dress appropriately: Balancing Exposure and Protection.

Dress appropriately when exposed to chilly temperatures. To avoid hypothermia or frostbite, strike a balance between cold exposure and the requirement for protective clothing. Layer garments to keep warm, then progressively expose more skin to cold stimuli as your tolerance grows.

- Practical Tip:

When exposed to chilly temperatures, use insulated clothes to preserve body heat. As you grow acclimated to the cold, gently modify your clothes to expose more flesh.

4. **Hydrate and Warm-Up: Helping the Body Respond**

Staying hydrated is critical during cold exposure, since dehydration can worsen the cold's effects on the body. Before cold exposure, engage in modest physical activity or warm-up activities to improve blood circulation and prepare the body for the event.

- Practical Tip:

Be well-hydrated before participating in cold exposure. Consider doing gentle workouts or dynamic stretches to warm up and increase circulation.

Using Heat for Metabolic Resilience: Embracing the Warmth Within

While cold exposure has advantages, heat exposure enhances metabolic resistance in distinct ways. Let's look at the benefits of embracing warmth and how heat can be a great tool for improving metabolic health.

1. Higher Energy Expenditure: The Thermogenic Effect of Heat

Heat exposure, whether in saunas or other hot places, increases energy consumption. This thermogenic action causes the body to try to remove heat, which burns calories. Regular heat exposure can help with weight control and metabolic health.

- Practical Tip

Incorporate sauna treatments or spend time in warm places to reap the thermogenic benefits of heat. Begin with shorter durations and progressively increase as your body adjusts.

2. Enhanced Cardiovascular Function: Heat Promotes Heart Health

Heat produces vasodilation, or the widening of blood vessels, which improves cardiovascular function. This impact improves blood flow, lowers blood pressure, and promotes cardiovascular health. Heat exposure can be especially useful for people who have cardiovascular problems.

- Practical Tip:

Incorporate heat exposure, such as saunas or heated baths. To guarantee your safety, see a healthcare expert, especially if you have any pre-existing cardiovascular conditions.

3. Enhanced Detoxification: Sweating Out Toxins.

Heat causes perspiration, which is a natural process that helps the body expel pollutants. Sweating during heat exposure can help with detoxification by releasing pollutants via the skin. This procedure helps the body's natural detoxification systems.

- Practical Tip:

Stay hydrated before and during hot exposure to help the sweating process. Consider sauna sessions or other sweat-inducing activities for cleansing.

4. Stress Relief and Relaxation: Heat for Mental Health

Heat exposure, particularly in the form of saunas or warm baths, improves relaxation and reduces tension. The relaxing impact of heat on the body extends to the mind, promoting mental well-being and lowering stress-related chemicals.

- Practical Tip

Incorporate heat exposure as a relaxing technique. Sauna sessions, warm baths, or spending time in warm locations can provide revitalizing experiences for both the body and mind.

Safe and Effective Practices for Heat Exposure: Embrace the Warmth

Similar to cold exposure, adding heat exposure into our daily routine necessitates a careful and progressive approach. Understanding individual tolerance, being hydrated, and being conscious of length and intensity are all important aspects of a safe and successful heat exposure practice.

1. Know Your Limits: Individualized Heat Practices

Individual heat tolerance varies depending on age, health state, and hydration levels. Begin with shorter times and lower temperatures, then gradually increase them as your body adjusts. Pay attention to symptoms of pain and adapt accordingly.

- Practical Tip

If you are new to heat exposure, begin with brief sessions in a sauna or warm setting. Pay attention to your body's reactions, and avoid continuous exposure until you've developed tolerance.

2. Stay Hydrated: Key to Heat Resilience

Hydration is essential during heat exposure to prevent dehydration and aid the body's cooling systems. Drink water before, during, and after heat exposure to keep fluids balanced and have a safe and happy experience.

- Practical Tip

Bring a water bottle to sauna sessions or other heat-related activities. Listen to your body's thirst cues and drink as needed.

3. Gradual Adaptation: Increasing Heat Resilience

Similar to cold exposure, progressive adaptation is critical for developing heat resilience. Give your body time to acclimate to greater temperatures and longer periods. To avoid heat-related concerns, try not to push yourself too hard.

- Practical Tip

Begin with lower temps and brief periods of heat exposure. Increase gradually as you feel more comfortable, paying close attention to your body's responses.

4. Cooling Strategies: Balancing Heat with Comfort

To ensure comfort, use cooling measures both during and after heat exposure. This might involve taking breaks to cool off, utilizing fans, or relaxing in a cold shower. Balancing heat with intervals of coolness improves the overall experience.

- Practical Tip:

Keep a cold cloth or water spray on hand during hot exposure. Take breaks to calm down and make sure that the whole experience is pleasurable.

Conclusion: Embracing Thermal Symphony for Metabolic Harmony

In conclusion, Chapter 9 has revealed the interesting relationship between temperature exposure and metabolic resilience. From the frigid grasp of cold to the comfortable warmth of heat, each element provides distinct advantages to our bodies.

Understanding the science of harnessing temperature exposure and applying safe and effective techniques enables us to harness the power of cold and heat for metabolic health. Whether it's stimulating brown adipose tissue with cold exposure or improving cardiovascular function with heat, the thermal symphony adds to general health.

As we include temperature exposure into our daily lives, let us approach it with curiosity, attention, and a desire for balance. The thermal symphony evolves into a harmonic dance that promotes metabolic resilience, increases energy expenditure, and adds to a vigorous and healthy lifestyle. So, let the thermal symphony begin: a voyage toward metabolic equilibrium, energy, and a life enriched by the embrace of both cold and warmth.

Chapter 10

Navigating the Grocery Store for Good Energy Foods

A Guide to Making Informed Decisions in the Aisles

Making decisions that match with our search for excellent energy and optimal metabolic health in today's hectic grocery store scene needs knowledge and purpose. Chapter 10 acts as a navigational aid, leading us through the aisles with tips on making educated decisions and choosing nutrient-dense products to power our bodies with vigor. Let's discover the mysteries of the grocery store and learn practical techniques for turning our shopping trip into a voyage toward high-energy foods.

Making Informed Choices in the Aisles: Understanding Food Labels and Marketing

1. Understanding Food Labels: Unveiling the Essentials

Food labels may be a maze of information, and understanding them is essential for making educated decisions. Key components to focus on are:

- Nutrition Facts: Look for the serving size, calorie count, and nutritional breakdown. Be aware of additional sugars, saturated fats, and salt.

GOOD ENERGY COOKBOOK: UNLEASHING THE POWER OF ENERGETIC LIVING

- Ingredients List: The components are presented in descending order of weight. Choose items that have entire, identifiable components and minimum additives.

- Allergy Information: If you are sensitive to or allergic to any allergens, look for warning labels.

- Expiry Dates: To ensure best quality, keep items within their freshness dates.

- Certification: Look for certifications such as USDA Organic, Non-GMO, or Heart-Healthy, which indicate certain quality criteria.

- Practical Tip

Take a minute to examine the labels, paying close attention to the nutritional content and ingredient list. Choosing items with less processed components promotes excellent energy.

2. Navigating Marketing Strategies: Beyond Hype

Food packaging sometimes includes appealing labels and marketing promises that may not necessarily correspond to nutritional value. Be aware of words like "low-fat," "low-calorie," and "natural," which can be deceptive. Instead, focus on the nutritional content and components.

- Natural versus Processed: The adjective "natural" does not necessarily indicate a product's healthfulness. Consider the nutritional profile and ingredient quality.

- Whole Foods vs Supplements: Opt for whole foods rather than supplements. Whole foods provide a variety of nutrients and synergistic chemicals.

- Local and Seasonal Options: Whenever possible, select local and seasonal food. These alternatives are often fresher and may include more nutrients.

- Practical Tip:
Look past marketing hype and showy brands. Choose based on the nutritional content and quality of the components.

3. Strategic Shopping: Plan for Success

Reading labels isn't the only way to navigate the grocery shop; strategic preparation is also required. Consider the following suggestions for a great shopping experience:

- Make a List: Plan your meals for the week and make a grocery list. This keeps you focused and prevents impulsive buying.

- Shop at the Perimeter: The store's perimeter often holds fresh vegetables, dairy, and protein sources. Spend additional time here to find nutrient-dense choices.

- Avoid Impulse Buying: Marketing strategies, such as displaying appealing things at eye level, might result in spontaneous purchases. Stick to your list and avoid making extraneous additions.

- Bulk Section Benefits: The bulk area allows you to purchase specific amounts of grains, nuts, and legumes, eliminating packaging waste and providing more cost-effective options.

- Practical Tip

Plan your shopping visits, shop with purpose, and avoid distractions to make strategic choices that include high-energy foods.

Tips for Selecting Nutrient-Dense Ingredients: Creating a Foundation for Good Energy Meal

1. Prioritize Whole Foods: The Essence of Nutrient Density.

Whole foods, in both raw and minimally processed forms, are the foundation of nutrient-dense nutrition. These foods are high in critical elements such vitamins, minerals, fiber, and antioxidants.

- fruits and vegetables: Aim to load your cart with a variety of bright veggies and fruits. These foods are rich in vitamins, minerals, and phytonutrients, all of which are necessary for good health.

- Whole Grain: Instead of refined carbohydrates, choose whole grains such as quinoa, brown rice, oats, and whole wheat. Whole grains include fiber, which improves digestion and offers sustained energy.

- Lean Protein: Use lean protein sources such poultry, fish, tofu, lentils, and eggs. Protein is essential for muscle repair, immunity, and satiety.

- healthy fats: Include sources of healthy fats including avocados, nuts, seeds, and olive oil. These fats improve brain function, hormone synthesis, and nutrient absorption.

- Practical Tip:
Fill your basket with a range of nutritious foods, including vegetables, fruits, whole grains, and lean meats, to ensure a nutrient-dense foundation.

2. Mindful Meat and Dairy Choices: Quality Counts

For people who consume meat and dairy, selecting high-quality selections is critical. Search for:

- Grass-fed and pasture-reared meat: These selections are often leaner and higher in omega-3 fatty acids than their traditionally reared equivalents.

- Organic, hormone-free dairy: Choose organic and hormone-free dairy products to minimize potential exposure to antibiotics and synthetic hormones.

- Sustainable Seafood: Choose sustainably produced seafood to encourage ethical fishing techniques and protect marine ecosystems.

- Plant-based alternatives: For more diversity and a lower environmental effect, try plant-based protein options like tofu, tempeh, and lentils.

- Practical Tip:

When purchasing meat and dairy products, consider quality, sustainability, and ethical methods.

3. Reduce Processed Foods: Added Sugars and Additives

Processed foods frequently have additional sugars, preservatives, and other ingredients that might lead to "bad energy" rather than "good energy." Be cautious about:

- Additional sugars: Check ingredient lists for hidden sugars that go by names like sucrose, high-fructose corn syrup, or agave nectar. Limiting added sugars improves metabolic health.

- artificial additives: Avoid items that include too many artificial additives, preservatives, and flavors. Choose meals with minimal ingredient lists.

- entire Snacking: Choose entire snacks such as fresh fruit, vegetables, nuts, or yogurt over excessively processed snack items. These solutions give lasting energy with no additional sugars.

- Practical Tip: Check labels for additional sugars and artificial ingredients. Choose whole, minimally processed snacks and meals.

4. Smart Carb Options: Embracing Complex Carbohydrates

Carbohydrates are an important source of energy, and eating the appropriate ones may help you stay energized. Opt for

- whole, unrefined carbohydrates: Choose whole grains such as brown rice, quinoa, and oats over refined alternatives. Whole, unprocessed carbohydrates provide greater fiber and minerals.

- Colorful Vegetables: Add a variety of bright veggies to your meals. These include complex carbohydrates as well as a wide range of vitamins and minerals.

- Legumes: Include legumes like beans, lentils, and chickpeas. They're high in fiber, protein, and complex carbs.

- Practical Tip

Consume complex carbs from entire food sources to boost energy levels and metabolic wellness.

.

Conclusion: Making Grocery Shopping a Positive Energy Experience

As we get to the end of Chapter 10, the grocery store turns from a simple shopping location to a wonderland of options for high-energy meals. We set out on a path of deliberate and educated decisions, armed with knowledge of how to read labels, navigate marketing methods, and choose nutrient-rich products.

Navigating the grocery shop for excellent energy meals is about more than just what gets into the basket; it's also about developing a stronger relationship with the food we eat. By emphasizing complete, nutrient-dense foods, being attentive of our choices, and laying the groundwork for high-energy meals, we may significantly improve our metabolic health.

So, let the grocery shop be a source of empowerment and sustenance. With each educated decision, we contribute to our total well-being, enjoying the path toward increased energy, vitality, and a better, more aware existence.

Chapter 11

Cooking Techniques to Preserve Nutritional Value

A Culinary Guide to Maximizing Good Energy

In the lovely domain of the kitchen, Chapter 11 opens as a gourmet guide, revealing the secrets of cooking techniques that not only tickle our taste senses but also maintain the nutritional content of our products. As we progress through this chapter, we'll look at how different cooking methods affect the nutrient content of our meals, as well as recipes and recommendations for incorporating healthy energy into our culinary creations.

Maximizing Nutrient Retention via Cooking Methods: Unraveling the Science of Cooking

1. Sautéing and stir-frying: Quick and Nutritious

Sautéing and stir-frying cook food quickly at high heat, keeping both texture and nutrition. Quick cooking durations reduce nutritional loss, making them perfect for veggies and lean meats.

- Practical Tip:
Combine a range of colorful veggies with lean meats. To add flavor, use spices and herbs rather than excessive oils or sauces.

2. Steaming: Gentle Cooking for Maximum Nutrition

Steaming is a mild cooking method that reduces nutritional loss. It includes cooking food with steam while keeping vitamins, minerals, and antioxidants. Suitable for veggies, seafood, and cereals.

- Practical Tip:

Vary the steam duration for different veggies to create the appropriate texture. For added flavor, squeeze in some lemon or herbs.

3. Roasting and Baking: Improving Flavors Without Losing Nutrients

Roasting and baking entail cooking food in an oven, resulting in caramelization and enhanced tastes. While some nutritional loss may occur, these procedures work well for root vegetables, fruits, and meats.

- Practical Tip

Roast various veggies with olive oil and seasonings. Baking whole grains adds texture and taste to recipes.

4. Grilling: Adding Flavor with a Hint of Char

Grilling adds a unique smokey taste to food while retaining its nutritious value. Marinating foods before grilling can improve taste and moisture while preventing the production of potentially hazardous chemicals.

- Practical Tip

Grill colorful veggies, lean meats, or vegan substitutes. Marinate with herbs, garlic, and citrus to increase flavor.

Ingredients include white fish fillets (cod, tilapia, or halibut), fresh herbs (parsley, dill, cilantro), and lemon slices.

- Salt and pepper.
- Olive Oil

Instructions: - Place fish fillets on parchment paper.

- Season with salt and pepper, then garnish with fresh herbs and lemon slices.
- Fold the parchment paper into bundles and seal the edges.
- Steam the fish until it is opaque and flakeable.

- Tip: Choose herbs according on your preferences. Serve with steamed veggies or quinoa for a healthful supper.

3. Roasted Vegetable Medley with Nature's Color Palette

Ingredients: - Mixed veggies (sweet potatoes, bell peppers, zucchini, cherry tomatoes) - Olive oil.

- Herbs: rosemary, thyme, oregano.
- Salt and pepper.

Instructions: - Toss veggies with olive oil, herbs, salt, and pepper. Roast veggies in the oven until soft and caramelized.

- Serve as a side dish, or combine with nutritious grains for a full dinner.

- Tip: Experiment with different herbal mixtures. Leftovers can be mixed into salads or grain bowls.

4. Grilled Citrus-Marinated Chicken Skewers: A Flavorful Delight.

Ingredients: - Cubed chicken breast.

- Marinade (orange juice, lime juice, garlic, cilantro, and olive oil).

- Skewer with bell peppers, onions, and cherry tomatoes.

Instructions: - Combine marinade ingredients and coat chicken cubes.

- Thread marinated chicken and veggies on skewers.

- Grill until the chicken is well cooked and the veggies are browned.

- Tip: Adjust marinade ingredients to your liking. Serve with a dish of quinoa or a fresh salad.

5. Hearty Lentil and Vegetable Soup: A Nutritious Bowl

Ingredients: - Green or brown lentils.

- Mix veggies (carrots, celery, onions, spinach) - Use low-sodium vegetable broth - Add herbs (thyme, bay leaves)

- Olive Oil

- Salt and pepper.

Instructions: - Sauté onions, carrots, and celery in olive oil until tender.

- Combine the lentils, veggies, broth, and herbs. Simmer until the lentils are soft.

- Season with salt and pepper, to taste.

- Tip: Batch cook for meal preparation. Freeze separate amounts for nutritious lunches.

6. Blanched Asparagus and Walnut Salad: A Fresh Side

Ingredients: - Fresh asparagus spears.

Toppings include toasted walnuts, lemon vinaigrette (lemon juice, olive oil, Dijon mustard), grated Parmesan cheese, and salt and pepper.

Instructions: - Blanch asparagus till brilliant green and slightly tender.
   - Toss blanched asparagus with toasted walnuts and lemon vinaig.

Combine vinaigrette, Parmesan, and season with salt and pepper.

   - Tip: Add herbs or honey to the vinaigrette for more flavor depth. This salad goes great with grilled chicken or fish.

7. Microwave-Baked Sweet Potatoes: A Quick and Nutritious Side Dish

Ingredients for this recipe are sweet potatoes, olive oil, salt, and optional cinnamon.

Instructions: - Pierce sweet potatoes with a fork and microwave until cooked.
   - Split open and sprinkle with olive oil.
   - Season with salt and cinnamon, if preferred.

   - Tip: Top with Greek yogurt and almonds for a well-balanced snack or side dish.

Conclusion: Infusing Each Meal with Good Energy

In Chapter 11, cooking goes beyond conventional preparation; it becomes a transforming act, a culinary symphony in which components work together to maintain their nutritious value. By learning diverse culinary techniques and combining nutrient-dense dishes, we not only delight our taste senses but also provide our bodies with vitality.

As you begin on your culinary adventure, keep in mind that each meal is a chance to bring positive energy into your life. Experiment with tastes, use a variety of products, and enjoy the satisfaction of producing meals that not only please the palate but also benefit your general health. Allow the kitchen to be your painting, and may each meal be a masterpiece of excellent energy, vigor, and pleasure.

Chapter 12:
Recipes for Good Energy

Crafting Culinary Delights for Every Meal

In the heart of Chapter 12, we start on a culinary journey, examining a selection of recipes precisely crafted to infuse every meal with excellent energy. This gastronomic trip takes place throughout the day, including breakfast, lunch, supper, and those pleasant times in between with snacks and desserts. Let us dig into the art of creating meals that not only satisfy our taste sensations but also fuel our bodies, guaranteeing that we stay energized from dawn to sunset.

Breakfast: Fueling Your Day Right—A Wholesome Start for Good Energy

1. Good Energy Oatmeal Bowl

Ingredients: - Rolled oats - Almond milk.

- Fresh berries (blueberries or strawberries) - Chia seeds

- Almond Butter

- Honey

Directions: - Cook rolled oats with almond milk.

 - Finish with fresh berries, chia seeds, almond butter, and honey.

- Tip: Choose your preferred toppings. Add nuts or seeds for added crunch and nutritional diversity.

2. Avocado and Egg Toast

Ingredients: - Whole grain bread - Ripe avocado.

To prepare, add a poached or fried egg, sliced cherry tomatoes, salt, and pepper.

Directions: - Toast whole grain bread.
  - Spread mashed avocado on toast.
  - Garnish with a poached or fried egg and sliced cherry tomatoes, then season with salt and pepper.

  - Tip: Experiment with several whole-grain bread types. Sprinkle with chili flakes for added taste.

3. Smoothie Bowl Delight

Ingredients: Frozen mixed berries, banana, and Greek yogurt.
Ingredients include spinach leaves, granola, and coconut flakes.

Directions: - Blend frozen berries, banana, and Greek yogurt until smooth.
  - Pour into a bowl and garnish with spinach leaves, oats, and coconut flakes.

  - Tip: To provide taste diversity, vary the smoothie components. Include a handful of vegetables for extra nutrition.

4. Quinoa Breakfast Bowl

Ingredients include cooked quinoa, almond milk, sliced kiwi, pomegranate seeds, chopped walnuts, and maple syrup.

To prepare, combine cooked quinoa with almond milk. Top with kiwi, pomegranate seeds, walnuts, and maple syrup.

- Tip: Substitute quinoa with another whole grain, such as farro or barley. Use seasonal fruits to ensure freshness.

Lunch: Energizing Midday Meals, Sustenance for the Afternoon Hustle**

1) Mediterranean Chickpea Salad

Ingredients include cooked chickpeas, halved cherry tomatoes, sliced cucumber, finely chopped red onion, crumbled feta cheese, kalamata olives, and olive oil and lemon dressing.

Instructions: - Mix chickpeas, cherry tomatoes, cucumber, red onion, feta cheese, and Kalamata olives.
- Drizzle with the olive oil and lemon dressing.

- Tip: Add more vegetables or grilled chicken for a heartier supper.

2. Quinoa and Vegetable Wrap

Ingredients include cooked quinoa, whole-grain wrap, hummus, spinach leaves, and roasted veggies (e.g., bell peppers, zucchini, eggplant).
- Feta cheese crumbled

Instructions: - Spread hummus on a whole grain wrap.
  - Add cooked quinoa, spinach leaves, roasted veggies, and crumbled feta cheese.
  - Roll into a wrap and slice.

  - Tip: Use a variety of bright veggies to create a visually pleasing and nutrient-dense wrap.

3. The Salmon and Avocado Bowl

Ingredients include grilled salmon fillet, cooked quinoa, and sliced avocado.
Edamame beans, steamed
- Thinly sliced radishes with soy-ginger dressing.

Instructions: - Place grilled fish atop cooked quinoa.
  - Arrange the sliced avocado, steaming edamame beans, and thinly sliced radishes.
  - Drizzle with the soy-ginger dressing.

  - Tip: Replace salmon with grilled chicken or tofu. Dressing can be adjusted to your liking.

4. Vegan Buddha Bowl

Ingredients: Cooked brown rice, roasted sweet potatoes, and sautéed greens.
To prepare, shred red cabbage, slice avocado, and drizzle with tahini dressing.

Instructions: - Place cooked brown rice in a bowl.
 - Combine the roasted sweet potatoes, sautéed kale, shredded red cabbage, and sliced avocado.
 - Drizzle with tahini dressing.

 - Tip: Experiment with different roasted veggies. To add texture, top with seeds or nuts.

Dinner: Nourishing Dinners for Sustained Vitality - Culinary Comfort for Evening Relaxation

1. Grilled Chicken and Quinoa Stuffed Bell Peppers.

Ingredients for this dish include half bell peppers, shredded grilled chicken, cooked quinoa, drained and rinsed black beans, corn kernels, and salsa.
- Shredded cheese.

Instructions: Combine grilled chicken, cooked quinoa, black beans, corn, and salsa.
 - Fill bell peppers with the mixture.
 - Sprinkle with shredded cheese and bake until it is melted and bubbling.

Tip: Add more vegetables to the filling or substitute ground turkey for the chicken.

2) Vegetarian Eggplant Lasagna

GOOD ENERGY COOKBOOK: UNLEASHING THE POWER OF ENERGETIC LIVING

Ingredients: - Eggplant cut lengthwise - Marinara sauce

Ingredients include ricotta cheese, spinach leaves, and shredded mozzarella cheese.

- Parmesan cheese, grated

Instructions: - Layer sliced eggplant with marinara sauce, ricotta cheese, spinach leaves, and mozzarella.

- Repeat layers and sprinkle with Parmesan.
- Bake till bubbling and golden.

- Tip: Add mushrooms or zucchini for more veggie deliciousness. To increase fiber, use whole-grain marinara sauce.

3. Shrimp and Broccoli Stir Fry

Ingredients: Peeled and deveined shrimp, broccoli florets, chopped bell peppers, and snow peas.

Ingredients include minced garlic and soy sauce.

Sesame oil

Instructions: Sauté shrimp in sesame oil until done.

- Add the broccoli, bell peppers, snow peas, and minced garlic.
- Stir-fry the veggies until crisp-tender, then add the soy sauce.

- Tip: Serve over brown or cauliflower rice for a low-carb alternative.

4. Lentil and Vegetable Curry.

Ingredients: - Cooked green or brown lentils

Ingredients: - Mixed veggies (carrots, bell peppers, and peas) - Coconut milk.

- Curry Powder

– Turmeric

Cilantro, chopped

Simmer cooked lentils and veggies in coconut milk.
- Stir in the curry powder and turmeric.
- Just before serving, garnish with chopped cilantro.

- Tip: Adjust the curry powder and turmeric to your liking. Serve over quinoa or full grain rice.

Snacks & Treats: Healthy Options for Any Time of Day—Guilt

-Free indulgences**

1. Homemade Trail Mix

Ingredients: - Mixed nuts (almonds, walnuts, and cashews).
- Dried fruits: apricots, cranberries, raisins
- Dark chocolate chunks.

Instructions: Combine nuts, dried fruits, and dark chocolate pieces.

- Divide into tiny bags for easy on-the-go snacking.

- Tip: Add your favorite nuts and dried fruits. For extra antioxidants, choose dark chocolate that has at least 70% cocoa.

2) Greek Yogurt Parfait

Ingredients: - Greek yogurt.
- Fresh berries (strawberries or blueberries) - Granola - Honey.

Instructions: - Combine Greek yogurt, fresh berries, and granola.
  - Drizzle with honey for extra sweetness.

- Tip: Experiment with various fruit and granola combinations. For a more flavorful experience, use flavored Greek yogurt.

3. Frozen banana bites

Ingredients for this recipe are sliced bananas and peanut butter.
- Dark chocolate melted

Directions: - Spread peanut butter on banana slices.
  - Dip in melted dark chocolate then freeze until hard.

- Tip: For added diversity, try almond or cashew butters. Store a batch in the freezer for a fast sweet treat.

4. Vegetable Sticks with Hummus

Ingredients include carrot sticks, cucumber spears, bell pepper strips, and hummus.

To make a healthy snack, arrange vegetable sticks on a dish and serve with hummus.

- Tip: Try different veggies, such as cherry tomatoes or celery. Make your own hummus to add a personal touch.

Conclusion: Creating a Culinary Symphony of Positive Energy

As we wrap off our culinary journey in Chapter 12, we have a collection of dishes designed to infuse every meal with excellent energy. From the vivid breakfast bowls that start our day to the hearty meals that provide evening relief, and the guilt-free snacks and pleasures in between, each recipe exemplifies the skill of balancing flavor and nutrition.

May these recipes inspire you to begin your culinary adventure, transforming each meal into a symphony of positive energy, vigor, and contentment. Experiment with ingredients, enjoy the joy of cooking, and relish the delicious tastes that not only satisfy your taste buds but also improve your entire health. Bon appétit!

Conclusion:

Embracing the Good Energy Lifestyle

A Journey to Empowered Health

As we come to the end of our transforming trip through the pages of "Good Energy: The Surprising Connection Between Metabolism and Limitless Health," it is time to reflect on Dr. Casey Means' profound insights and practical knowledge. The trip has been transformative, revealing the enigmatic relationship between metabolism and general health, opening the door for a paradigm change in how we approach well-being.

The Essence of the Healthy Energy Lifestyle:

At its foundation, the Good Energy Lifestyle is a comprehensive approach to health that defies conventional knowledge. It's a way of living based on the concept that our metabolic function is the key to breaking free from common health problems like depression, anxiety, and heart disease. The key is to understand and optimize the body's ability to generate and use energy efficiently, which is the cornerstone of healthy energy.

Key Takeaways for the Good Energy Journey:

1. Metabolism Unveiled; The tour began by explaining the complicated workings of metabolism. From the fundamentals of metabolic function to its significant impact on our health and well-being, we discovered that practically every health problem is linked to how well our cells make and use energy.

2. Nutrition as a Powerhouse: The influence of nutrition on cellular energy was highlighted, highlighting the importance of nutrients in supporting optimal energy production. Dr. Means assisted us in creating balanced meals that act as sustainable energy sources, refuting nutritional fallacies, and providing concepts relevant to a variety of lifestyles, whether carnivorous or vegan.

3. Navigating Dietary Choices: Chapter 3 illuminated the characteristics of "bad energy" foods, assisting us in detecting and minimizing detrimental dietary choices. With this knowledge, readers learned how to make educated decisions, such as avoiding foods that disturb metabolic health and lead to life-threatening diseases.

4. Monitoring and Adjustment: Chapter 4 focused on the practical aspects of monitoring metabolic health through food, providing biomarkers as instruments for assessing nutritional status. Dr. Means allowed us to track our progress, make educated dietary changes, and take charge of our health.

5. Creating a Good Energy Meal Plan: The adventure continued to Chapter 5, where we learnt the skill of creating a four-week diet plan for maximum health. The emphasis was on diversity and balance, offering a comprehensive approach to fueling the body for long-term performance.

6. The Principles of Good Energy Eating: Chapter 6 debunked nutritional misconceptions and ideologies, dispelling the uncertainty around food choices. We accepted six lifetime eating principles that apply to every dietary preference, establishing the groundwork for long-term and sustainable health.

7. Sleep, Circadian Rhythm, and Metabolism: Chapter 7 explored the critical relationships between sleep, circadian rhythm, and metabolism. Practical ways were revealed to improve sleep quality and regularity, hence strengthening the body's capacity to sustain high energy levels.

8. Integrating Movement and Exercise: In Chapter 8, the emphasis switched to the importance of mobility and exercise in metabolic health. Readers were advised to engage in ordinary activities that boost physical activity and to develop a balanced exercise program to support overall wellbeing.

9. Advantages of Temperature Exposure: Chapter 9 looked at the advantages of using cold and heat for metabolic resilience. Safe and practical procedures were described, allowing readers to use temperature exposure to improve their overall health.

10. Navigating the Grocery Store: Chapter 10 turned the grocery store from a basic shopping location to a wonderland of high-energy food options. Readers learned about making educated decisions, choosing nutrient-dense products, and turning grocery shopping into a thoughtful and empowered experience.

Empowering readers to take control:

As we embrace the Good Energy Lifestyle, we realize that optimal health is within grasp. The book acts as a guide, providing readers with knowledge and tools to help them take charge of their health journey. Dr. Casey Means' innovative research and practical insights enable us to:

- **Understanding Our Body:** Readers are equipped with information about metabolism and its significant influence, allowing them to comprehend their bodies at the molecular level. This understanding helps as a guidepost for making sound decisions regarding lifestyle, diet, and general well-being.

- **Make Informed Decisions:** The book offers more than just facts; it also gives a road map for making educated decisions. Whether it's choosing nutrient-dense meals, tracking biomarkers, or including temperature exposure, readers have the tools they need to manage their health journeys.

- **Adopt Sustainable Practices:** The book's ideas are long-term practices that may be incorporated into daily living, rather than fast remedies. From food planning to physical activity, the Good Energy Lifestyle is a journey rather than a destination, delivering long-term effects.

- **Transform lifestyle habits:** Readers are inspired to change their living habits after learning about the connections between sleep, circadian rhythm, and metabolism. Practical ways for improving sleep and incorporating activity into daily activities lay the path for long-term vitality.

- **How to Confidently Navigate the Grocery Store:** Chapter 10 provides a step-by-step plan for transforming the grocery store into a hub for healthy energy foods. Readers are advised to study labels, understand marketing strategies, and choose substances that promote their general well-being.

Conclusion: A Call to Action for Lifelong Well-being

As we complete this educational trip through "Good Energy," we are not just closing a book but also beginning a new chapter in our life. The Good Energy Lifestyle is a call to action, asking readers to embark on a path of lifetime well-being.

By adopting the ideas stated in the book, readers go on a transforming journey in which each decision adds to the development of positive energy. The journey is about development, not perfection, and about empowerment rather than constraint. It is a dedication to understanding, nourishing, and maximizing the body's extraordinary ability for vitality.

In the enormous fabric of our lives, health is a thread that runs through every moment. The Good Energy Lifestyle provides a compass, helping us to make choices that honor our bodies, boost our energy, and contribute to a life of vitality and well-being.

As you begin this new chapter, remember that you have the ability to improve your health. Accept the Good Energy Lifestyle, arm yourself with information, and go on a journey where each day is a chance to nourish your body, mind, and soul. May your journey be full of positive energy, resilience, and the joy of living well.

Glossary of Key Terms:

A Layperson's Guide to Understanding Good Energy and Metabolic Health

In the investigation of "Good Energy: The Surprising Connection Between Metabolism and Limitless Health," a slew of concepts have been presented, each playing an important part in unlocking the secrets of metabolic health. This dictionary attempts to give a thorough and user-friendly introduction to these major concepts, allowing readers to navigate the complicated terrain of health and well-being with ease and confidence.

1. Metabolism (Layman's Explanation)

Metabolism functions similarly to our body's engine. It refers to the processes that transform the food and beverages we consume into energy. This energy powers everything our bodies do, from breathing to running a marathon.

2. Biomarkers: -

Explanation by Layman: Biomarkers are tiny signals in our bodies. They are measurable indications that can help us determine how effectively our bodies are working. In the framework of "Good Energy," biomarkers are utilized to evaluate our metabolic health and highlight areas for improvement.

3. Nutrients:

- Explanation by Layman Nutrients are the basic building components contained in the food we consume. They contain vitamins, minerals, proteins, lipids, and carbs, which are required for our bodies to function effectively.

4. Good Energy:

- Explanation by Layman: Good energy is the high-quality fuel that our bodies require to flourish. It results from consuming nutritious meals and leading a healthy lifestyle. When our cells are charged with healthy energy, we feel energized, aware, and prepared to face life's difficulties.

5. Bad Energy Foods

- Explanation by Layman: Bad energy foods are the villains of our diet. These are frequently processed and sugary meals, which can harm our metabolic health. Identifying and reducing these foods is critical for avoiding long-term health problems.

6. Circadian Rhythm:

- Explanation by Layman The circadian rhythm is our body's internal clock, which governs a variety of biological activities such as sleep-wake cycles, hormone synthesis, and metabolism. It's like a natural timetable that allows our bodies to perform effectively.

7. Biomarkers of Aging:

- Explanation by Layman Biomarkers of aging are indicators in the body that indicate how well we are aging. By tracking these signals, we can age gracefully and stay healthy.

8. Macronutrients:

- Explanation by Layman: Macronutrients are the major components of our food, including proteins, fats, and carbs. These give our bodies with a significant quantity of energy and important nutrients.

9. Micronutrients:

- Explanation by Layman Vitamins and minerals are examples of micronutrients, which act as supporting characters. Although in modest numbers, they perform critical roles in a variety of body activities, promoting general health.

10. Sleep Hygiene:
- Explanation by Layman Sleep hygiene refers to excellent behaviors that encourage restful sleep. It entails developing a suitable sleep environment, adhering to a consistent sleep schedule, and implementing activities that promote restful evenings.

11. Resilience:
- Explanation by Layman; Resilience refers to our body's capacity to recover and adapt to adversities. Building metabolic resilience entails reinforcing our bodies against stresses, allowing them to remain balanced and healthy.

12. Whole Foods:
- Explanation by Layman Whole foods are foods in their original, unadulterated form. They are high in nutrients and have less additives than processed meals. Focusing on complete foods is an important factor for creating excellent energy.

13. Inflammation:
- Explanation by Layman Inflammation is the body's reaction to damage or illness. Chronic inflammation, on the other hand, has been linked to a variety of health concerns. Adopting a lifestyle that decreases chronic inflammation is critical for general health.

14. Free Radicals:

- Explanation by Layman Free radicals are renegade chemicals in the body that can harm cells. Certain foods include antioxidants, which neutralize free radicals and aid to protect our cells.

15. Homeostasis:

- Explanation by Layman Homeostasis functions as the body's thermostat, ensuring internal equilibrium. It ensures that our bodies work within a small range to promote good health.

16. Microbiome:

- Explanation by Layman The microbiome is the population of billions of bacteria that live in our stomach. This "gut flora" has a significant impact on digestion, nutrient absorption, and general health.

17. Insulin Resistance:

- Explanation by Layman Insulin resistance happens when:

Our cells may not respond properly to insulin, a hormone that controls blood sugar. It's like a lock-and-key situation, resulting in high blood sugar levels and an increased risk of health problems.

18. Intermittent Fasting:

- Explanation by Layman: Intermittent fasting is an eating habit that alternates between periods of eating and fasting. It's similar to giving our digestive system a rest, encouraging metabolic flexibility and possible health advantages.

19. Ketosis:

- Explanation by Layman Ketosis is a condition in which the body uses fat as fuel instead of carbs. It's like transitioning from gasoline to a more efficient and sustainable energy source.

20. Thermogenesis:

- Explanation by Layman: Thermogenesis is the body's method for creating heat. It functions similarly to the body's natural heater, and activities such as exercise and exposure to cold can increase thermogenesis, hence aiding metabolism.

21. Mindful Eating:

- Explanation by Layman: Mindful eating entails paying attention to what, when, and how we consume. It's like savoring every taste, cultivating a positive relationship with food, and avoiding overeating.

22. Macronutrient Ratio:

- Explanation by Layman The macronutrient ratio refers to the proportions of proteins, lipids, and carbohydrates in our diet. Finding the proper balance based on individual demands is critical for maintaining metabolic health.

23. Prebiotics:

- Explanation by Layman Prebiotics are like food for the beneficial bacteria in our stomach. They are non-digestible fibers present in some foods that aid in the formation of good gut flora.

24. Postbiotics:

- Explanation by Layman Postbiotics are metabolites created by helpful intestinal microorganisms. These byproducts can have a good impact on our health, adding to overall wellbeing.

25. Mind-Body Connection: - Explanation by Layman: The mind-body connection stresses the close relationship between mental and physical wellness. Adopting behaviors that create harmonious connections improves general well-being.

25. Epigenetics:

- Explanation by Layman: Epigenetics studies how our lifestyle and environment affect our genes. It's like a ballet between nature and nurture, demonstrating how our decisions influence our genetic expression.

26. Sustainability:

- Explanation by Layman Food sustainability entails making decisions that are beneficial to both our own and the planet's health. It's a win-win scenario that promotes long-term well-being and environmental protection.

27. Mindful Movement:

- Explanation by Layman* Mindful movement is the practice of incorporating purposeful and joyful physical activity into one's daily life. It's like incorporating exercise into our daily routine in a way that feels good and is sustainable.

28. Thermic Effect of Food (TEF):

- Explanation by Layman TEF is the amount of energy expended by our bodies to digest, absorb, and assimilate nutrients from the food we ingest. It's similar to the calorie-burning activity that occurs before and after a meal.

29. Bioindividuality:

- Explanation by Layman: Bioindividuality acknowledges that everyone is unique, and there is no one-size-fits-all solution to health. It's similar to accepting bespoke solutions tailored to individual requirements and tastes.

Conclusion: Navigating the Path to Wellbeing with Confidence

As we finish our trip through the glossary of essential terminology, we've armed ourselves with a toolbox of comprehension. From the complexities of metabolism to the importance of mindful eating and the marvels of the microbiome, each phrase contributes significantly to the great symphony of well-being.

With this information, readers may confidently follow the route to optimal energy and metabolic health. The dictionary serves as a beacon, illuminating sometimes difficult topics in ways that are understandable to the average person. As we accept these concepts, may we find empowerment in our understanding, clarity in our choices, and the courage to start on a lifetime quest for maximum health and unlimited well-being.

PLEASE HELP BY LEAVING REVIEW ON AMAZON
PLEASE, FOR THIS IT WILL REACH MANY MORE
READERS THAT WILL NEED IT

Made in the USA
Middletown, DE
17 October 2024